EXAMINATION AND TREATMENT METHODS IN DOGS AND CATS

Examination and Treatment Methods in Dogs and Cats

2nd edition

Christian F. Schrey

Translated by Heidi Joeken

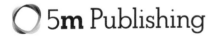 5m Publishing

First published 2014

Authorised translation of the second German language edition

Christian F. Schrey, Untersuchungs- und Behandlungsmethoden bei Hund und Katze

Published by
5M Publishing Ltd,
Benchmark House,
8 Smithy Wood Drive,
Sheffield, S35 1QN, UK
Tel: +44 (0) 1234 81 81 80
www.5mpublishing.com

A catalogue record for this book is available from the British Library

ISBN 978-1-910455-16-6

Book layout by Florence Production Ltd, Stoodleigh, Devon, UK

Printed by Replika Press Pvt. Ltd, India

Illustrations by Schattauer

First published 2014

Dr. med. vet. Christian F. Schrey MS, MRCVS
Tierarztpraxis am Olivaer Platz Lietzenburger Straße 107
10707 Berlin www.vet-berlin.de
VetSchrey@t-online.de

To the three bright sparks
in my life, giving me perspective:
Sabiene, Noona and Philipp

Acknowledgements

Every day I use this book at least once to check upon or find something quickly. It looks battered, discoloured and well-thumbed and lives on a shelf in our practice.

It is with great delight that I found this book in veterinary practices around the world in exactly this condition.

My thanks go to Dr Sabine Schmidt, Pippo Farnedi, Dr Karl-Heinz Kirschstein, Oliver Cescotti, Nicolai Hildebrand, Dr Johann Homm, Dr Frank-Ullrich Hügel, Alexander Hüttig, Dr Kirsten Peters, Schwester Andrea from the hospital Waldfriede in Berlin, Dr Bernhard Sörensen, Hayden Yates and to the staff at Schattauer Publishers, in particular to Dr Wulf Bertram and Dr Petra Mülker. With their help we managed to create a handbook for the most often required working techniques in the daily lives of the small animal practitioner.

Dr Med Vet Christian F. Schrey
Berlin, August 2013

Contents

Part I
Examination Methods

1 General Examination Methods

Restraining the Patient

Indication

- Immobilisation of the patient prior to examination and treatment

Restraining Methods in the Dog

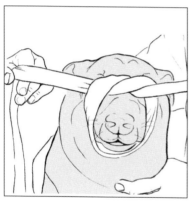

Fig 1.1 Mouth sling (step 1)

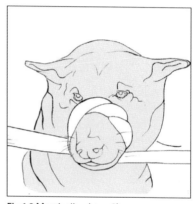

Fig 1.2 Mouth sling (step 2)

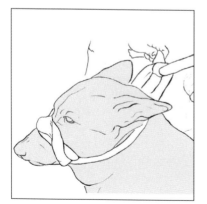

Fig 1.3 Mouth sling (step 3)

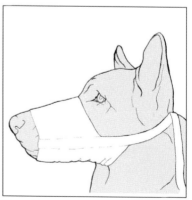

Fig 1.4 Muzzle

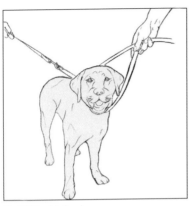

Fig 1.5 Double lead

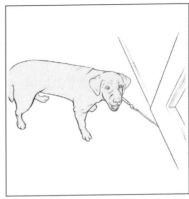

Fig 1.6 Feeding the lead under a door

Method

- **Mouth sling**
    - Place a prepared gauze loop over the muzzle
    - Cross over the ties underneath the throat
    - Tie the ends behind the ears

- **Muzzle**
    - Choose the appropriate size
    - To be fitted by the owner
    - Close the ties behind the ears

- **Double lead**
    - Immobilisation of the dog between two leads

- **Feeding lead under door**
    - Owner leaves the room with dog on the lead
    - Closure of the door between owner and dog
    - Lead is fed under the door and pulled tight (take care)

Restraining Methods in the Cat

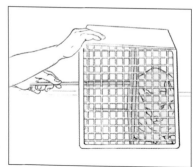

Fig 1.7 Crush cage

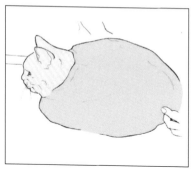

Fig 1.8 Strait jacket or sack

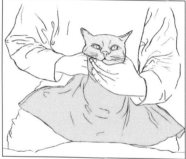

Fig 1.9 Towel

Method

- **Crush cage**
  - Preparation: assemble the pushing wall and the rod
  - Tip the cat out of its transport box into the crush cage (cover the sides with towels)
  - Close the cage door in a coordinated manner
  - Restrain the cat between the mobile pushing and side wall

- **Strait jacket or sac**

- **Towel**
  - Suitable for manipulation by the owners
  - Immobilise the cat between your knees and closed ankles while kneeling
  - Place the towel around the neck and front legs of the cat

Transport

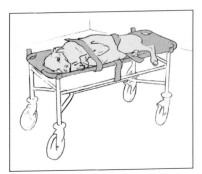

Fig 1.10 Trolley with stretcher

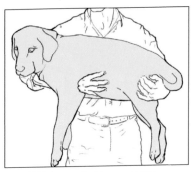

Fig 1.11 Being carried by one person

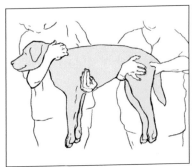

Fig 1.12 Being carried by two people

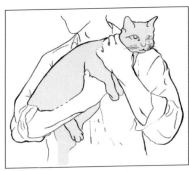

Fig 1.13 Carrying of a relaxed cat

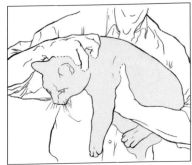

Fig 1.14 Carrying a cat safely

Lifting

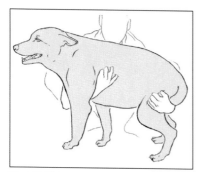

Fig 1.15 Lifting by one person

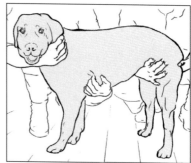

Fig 1.16 Lifting by two people

Holding the dog

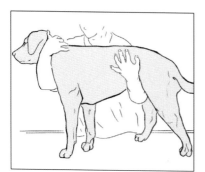

Fig 1.17 Holding while the dog is standing (one person)

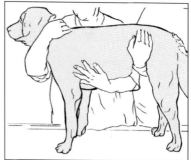

Fig 1.18 Holding while the dog is standing (two people)

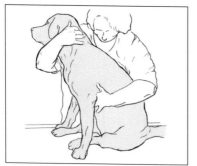

Fig 1.19 Holding while the dog is sitting

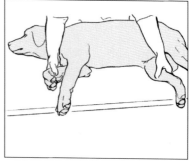

Fig 1.20 Holding while the dog is in lateral recumbency

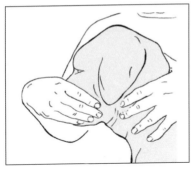

Fig 1.21

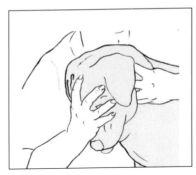

Fig 1.22

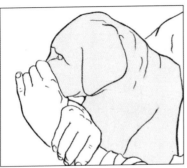

Fig 1.23 Holding whilst examining the ear

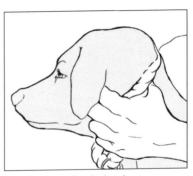

Fig 1.24 Restraining the head

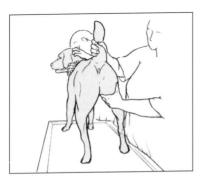

Fig 1.25 Holding while examining the perineum

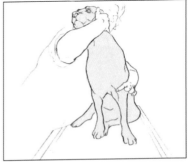

Fig 1.26 Holding for blood sampling (standing or sitting)

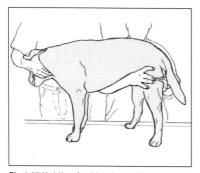

Fig 1.27 Holding for blood sampling (standing)

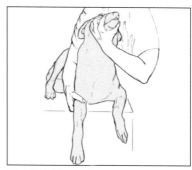

Fig 1.28 Holding for blood sampling (lying down)

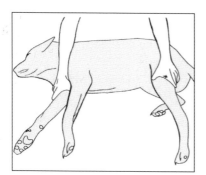

Fig 1.29 Holding for Blood Sampling (Lying down)

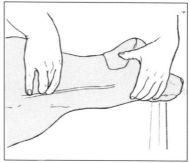

Fig 1.30 Holding for Jugular Blood Sampling (Lying down)

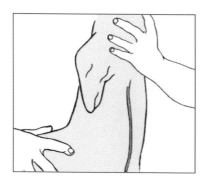

Fig 1.31 Holding for Jugular Blood Sampling (Standing)

Holding the Cat

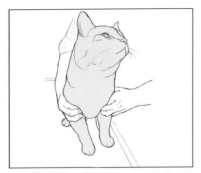

Fig 1.32 Holding while the cat is standing

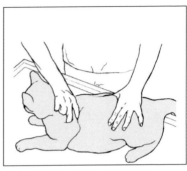

Fig 1.33 Holding in sternal position

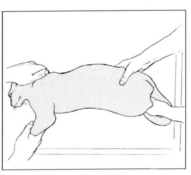

Fig 1.34 Holding in lateral recumbency
(two people)

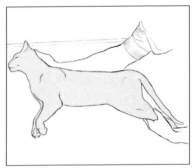

Fig 1.35 Holding in lateral recumbency
(one person)

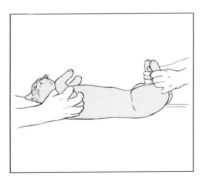

Fig 1.36 Holding in dorsal position
(two people)

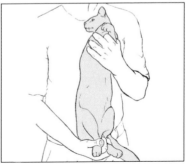

Fig 1.37 Holding in dorsal position
(one person)

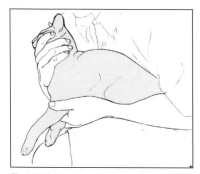

Fig 1.38 Holding for blood sampling (cephalic vein)

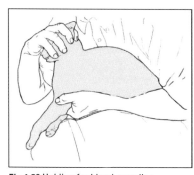

Fig 1.39 Holding for blood sampling (cephalic vein)

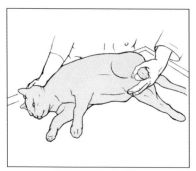

Fig 1.40 Holding for blood sampling (back leg)

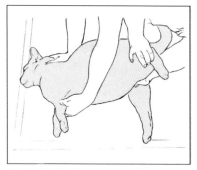

Fig 1.41 Holding for blood sampling (back leg)

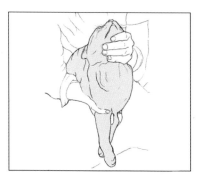

Fig 1.42 Holding for jugular blood sampling

Lying Down

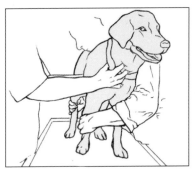

Fig 1.43 Lift and rotate into lateral position

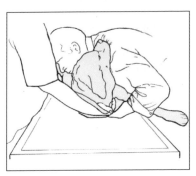

Fig 1.44 Lay the patient down gently on his side

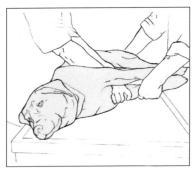

Fig 1.45 Readjust the holding hands to keep the patient down

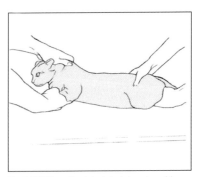

Fig 1.46 Lift and rotate into lateral position

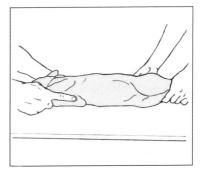

Fig 1.47 Lay the patient down gently

Blood Sampling: Venous Blood Sampling

Indication

- Full in-house or external laboratory blood investigation
- Transfusion

Venous Blood Sampling in the Dog

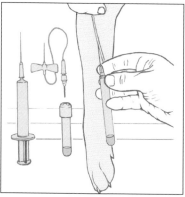

Fig 1.48 Puncture of the cephalic vein of the forelimb (1)

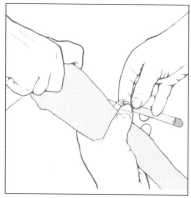

Fig 1.49 Puncture of the cephalic vein of the forelimb (2)

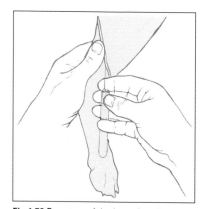

Fig 1.50 Puncture of the lateral saphenous vein (1)

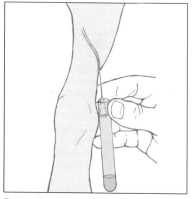

Fig 1.51 Puncture of the lateral saphenous vein (2)

Venous Blood Sampling in the Cat

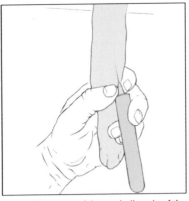

Fig 1.52 Puncture of the cephalic vein of the forelimb (1)

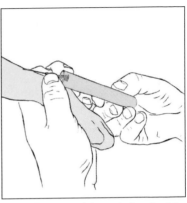

Fig 1.53 Puncture of the cephalic vein of the forelimb (2)

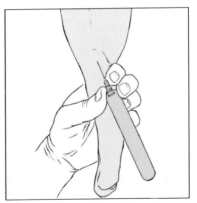

Fig 1.54 Puncture of the medial saphenous vein (1)

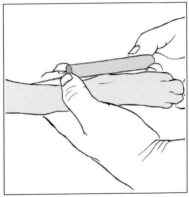

Fig 1.55 Puncture of the medial saphenous vein (2)

Method

- **Preparation**
    - Position of the patient: standing (dog); sitting/sternal (cat)
    - Separate/clip fur
    - Disinfect skin

    Venous stasis (manual/tourniquet)
    - Accessible veins for blood sampling in the dog
    - Cephalic vein of the forelimb
    - Lateral saphenous vein (external jugular vein)

    Accessible veins for blood sampling in the cat
    - Cephalic vein of the forelimb
    - Medial saphenous vein
    - External jugular vein

- **Technique**

    Fixation of the vein
    - Method 1: between thumb and middle finger
    - Method 2: lateral fixation with thumb

    Venous puncture
    - Nearly tangential puncture through the skin and venous wall
    - Further insertion of the cannula into the venous lumen
    - Fixation of the cannula between thumb and middle finger of the left hand

    Blood taking
    - Allow the blood to drop into blood tubes
    - Close the blood tubes and swill gently (EDTA/Heparin/Citrate)
    - Release the venous stasis
    - Remove the cannula and apply pressure with a swab
    - Light dressing/swab cover

Complications

- Paravascular malpuncture
- Haematoma
- Thrombophlebitis
- Air embolism

Blood Sampling: Arterial Blood Sampling

Indication

- Blood gas analysis (BGA)

Arterial Blood Sampling in the Dog

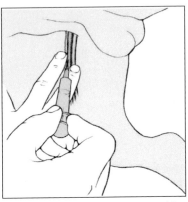

Fig 1.56 Puncture of the femoral artery (1)

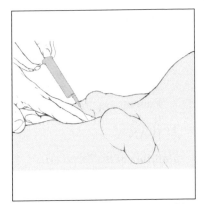

Fig 1.57 Puncture of the femoral artery (2)

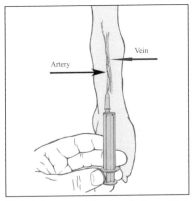

Fig 1.58 Puncture of the dorsal artery of the foot

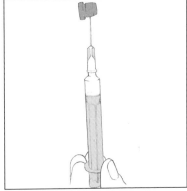

Fig 1.59 Airtight closure of the syringe

Method

- **Preparation**

    - Flush a syringe with heparin
    - Position of patient: lateral recumbency
    - Clip fur and disinfect skin

- **Technique**

    Palpation of the pulse
    - Fixation of artery
    - Fixation between the index and middle finger

    Puncture of the femoral artery
    - Syringe with attached cannula
    - Puncture the skin and arterial wall while slightly aspirating
      (c. 45°) until bright red pulsating blood flows in
    - IVAN (inside – vein – artery – nerve)

    Puncture of the dorsal artery of the foot
    - Syringe with attached cannula
    - Puncture the skin and arterial wall whilst slightly aspirating
      (c. 20°) until bright red pulsating blood flows in
    - Dorsal superficial artery is distal end of the hock slightly medial of
      the midline

    Blood sampling
    - Remove the cannula and apply pressure with swab
    - Compression (c. 5 min)
    - Light dressing/swab cover

- **Sample processing**

    - Removal of air bubbles
    - Puncture of a rubber bung with the cannula for airtight closure
    - Immediate processing of blood sample

Complications

- Paravascular malpuncture
- Accidental puncture of the femoral vein (dark blood, no pulsation)
- Damage to the femoral nerve
- Haematoma/abscess

2 Sample processing

Blood Sample

Indication

- Processing in order to send to external laboratory
- Processing for in-house analysis on site

Blood Smear (EDTA Tube)

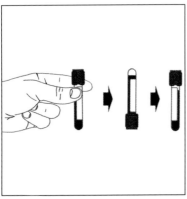

Fig 2.1 Swill EDTA tube gently after obtaining the sample

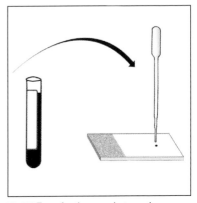

Fig 2.2 Transfer the sample to a microscope slide

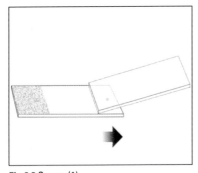

Fig 2.3 Smear (1)

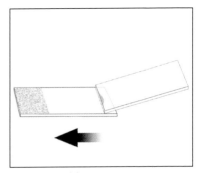

Fig 2.4 Smear (2)

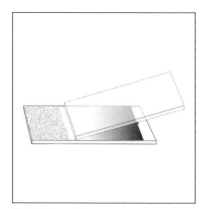

Fig 2.5 Smear (3)

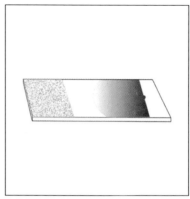

Fig 2.6 Leave the sample to dry

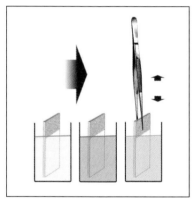

Fig 2.7 Fixate and stain

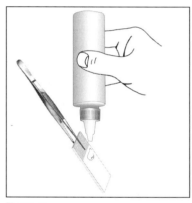

Fig 2.8 Rinse

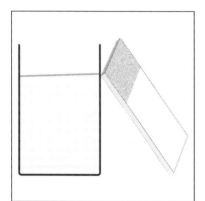

Fig 2.9 Dry

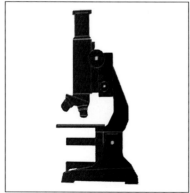

Fig 2.10 Microscopic examination

Serum Tube

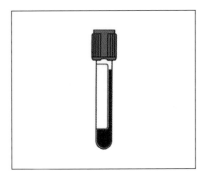

Fig 2.11 Leave the tube for 15–30 min

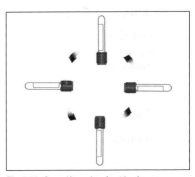

Fig 2.12 Centrifugation (c. 10 min. at 3,000 rpm)

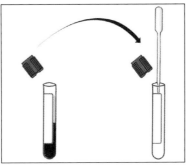

Fig 2.13 Pipette the serum off

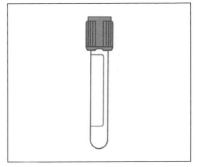

Fig 2.14 Blood chemistry analysis

Blood Sample: EDTA Tube

- **Technique**
    - Swill the tube gently after obtaining sample
    - Measure the blood glucose immediately
    - Differential blood count
    - Haematological laboratory investigation

Blood Sample: Differential Blood Count

- **Technique**
    - Transfer one drop of EDTA-blood onto a microscope slide
    - Approach the drop of blood with a cover slide (30–45°)
    - Push the cover slide after contact with the drop of blood swiftly along the microscope slide
    - Leave the smear to dry
    - Fixate and stain the smear
    - Rinse with water/distilled water
    - Leave the smear to dry in a tilted position
    - Perform a microscopic examination

Blood Sample: Serum Tube

- **Technique**
    - Leave the tube for 15–30 min at room temperature
    - Centrifugation for c. 10 min at 3,000 rpm
    - Pipette the serum off
    - Blood chemistry analysis

Complications

- Haemolysis
- Microthrombi

Paracentesis

Indication

- Thoracocentesis, Pericardiocentesis, Abdominocentesis, Tracheobronchial lavage, Nasal flush, Arthrocentesis, Cerebrospinal fluid puncture, CSF tap

Paracentesis

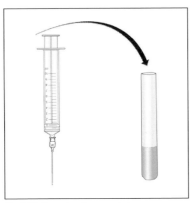

Fig 2.15 Transfer the sample into a test tube

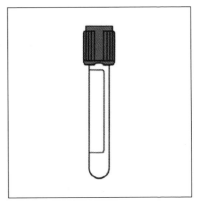

Fig 2.16 Dispatch the sample for laboratory analysis

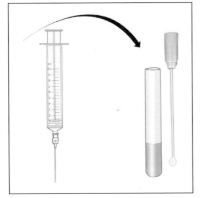

Fig 2.17 Transfer the sample into a culture tube for bacteriological examination

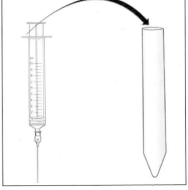

Fig 2.18 Transfer the sample into a centrifugation tube for cytological examination of sediment

Paracentesis: Examination of Sediment

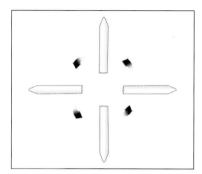

Fig 2.19 Centrifugation (c. 10 min at 3,000 rpm)

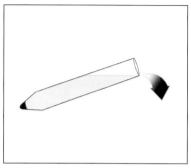

Fig 2.20 Decant the supernatant fluid

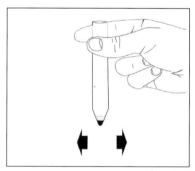

Fig 2.21 Plump up the sediment

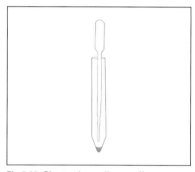

Fig 2.22 Pipette the sediment off

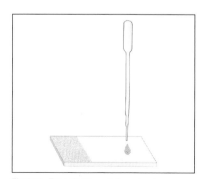

Fig 2.23 Transfer the sediment onto a microscope slide

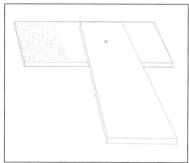

Fig 2.24 Smear (1)

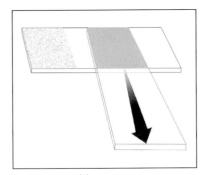

Fig 2.25 Smear (2)

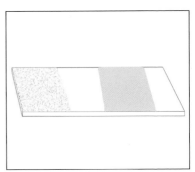

Fig 2.26 Dry

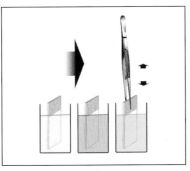

Fig 2.27 Fixate and stain

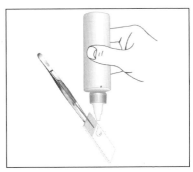

Fig 2.28 Rinse

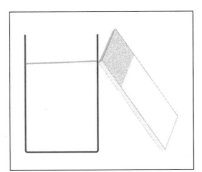

Fig 2.29 Dry

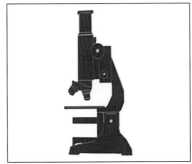

Fig 2.30 Microscopic examination

Method

- **Technique: examination of the sediment**

  - Transfer the sample into a pointed centrifugation tube
  - Centrifugation (c. 10 min at 3,000 rpm)
  - Decant the supernatant fluid
  - Plump up the sediment
  - Pipette the sediment off and transfer it onto a microscope slide
  - Make a smear
  - Dry the smear
  - Fixate and stain the smear
  - Rinse the smear with water/distilled water
  - Dry the smear in tilted position
  - Perform a microscopic examination

Fine Needle Aspiration Biopsy

Indication

- Tumour biopsy, Lymph node biopsy, Liver biopsy, Bone marrow biopsy, Prostate biopsy

Fine Needle Aspiration Biopsy

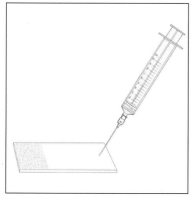

Fig 2.31 Transfer the sample to a microscope slide

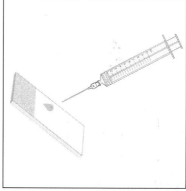

Fig 2.32 Syringe/spray sample onto a microscope slide (bone marrow)

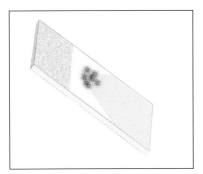

Fig 2.33 Let the blood run off (bone marrow)

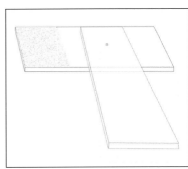

Fig 2.34 Smear (1)

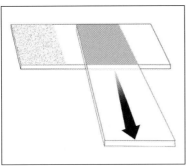

Fig 2.35 Smear (2)

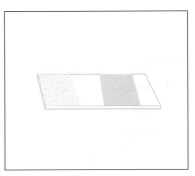

Fig 2.36 Dry

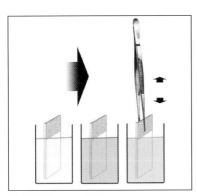

Fig 2.37 Fixate and stain

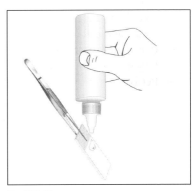

Fig 2.38 Rinse

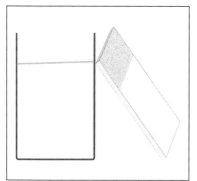

Fig 2.39 Dry

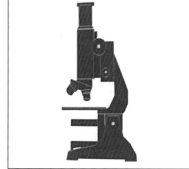

Fig 2.40 Microscopic examination

Method

- **Technique**

    - Transfer the sample onto a microscope slide

    Bone marrow
    - Spray the bone marrow out of the syringe onto a tilted microscope slide
    - Let the blood run off
    - Make a smear
    - Dry the smear
    - Fixate and stain the smear
    - Rinse the smear with water/distilled water
    - Dry the smear in a tilted position
    - Perform a microscopic examination

Tissue Sample (Biopsy)

Indication

- Skin punch biopsy, Tru-cut-organ/tumour biopsy, Endoscopic biopsy

Tissue Sample

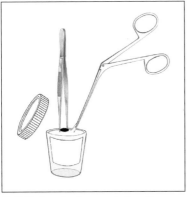

Fig 2.41 Transfer the sample from the biopsy forceps

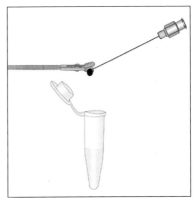

Fig 2.42 Transfer the sample from the endoscopy forceps

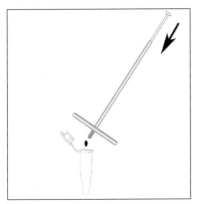

Fig 2.43 Transfer the sample from the bone biopsy needle

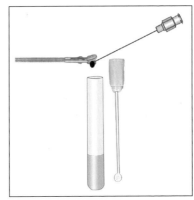

Fig 2.44 Transfer the sample into a culture tube

Tissue Sample: Cytological Preparation

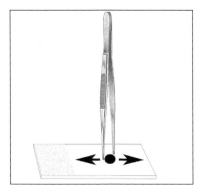

Fig 2.45 Cytological impression smear

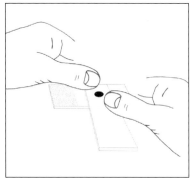

Fig 2.46 Cytological crushing preparation

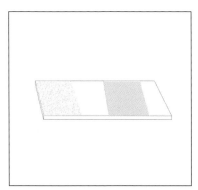

Fig 2.47 Dry

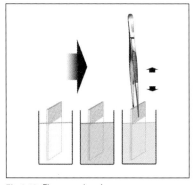

Fig 2.48 Fixate and stain

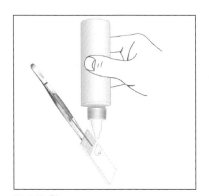

Fig 2.49 Rinse

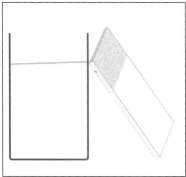

Fig 2.50 Dry

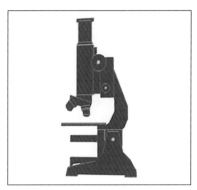

Fig 2.51 Microscopic examination

Histology

• **Technique**

Tissue biopsy
- Transfer the tissue sample into fixative solution (neutral buffered 4 per cent formaldehyde solution)

Muscle biopsy
- Place one muscle sample (fixated lengthwise on a wooden spatula) into a neutral buffered 4 per cent formaldehyde solution
- Place a further muscle sample into a phosphate buffered 5 per cent gluteraldehyde-solution (chilled at 4°C)

Bone Biopsy
- Transfer the bone sample with a moistened gauze into an Eppendorf tube (usually without fixation medium)

Cytology

• **Technique**
- Make an impression smear/crushing preparation
- Dry the sample
- Fixate and stain the sample
- Rinse the sample with water/distilled water
- Dry the sample in a tilted position
- Perform a microscopic examination

Microbiology

• **Technique**
- Transfer the tissue sample into a culture tube
- Dispatch the sample

Swab Sample

Indication

- Nasal/pharyngeal/tracheal/conjunctival/skin/ear canal/vaginal/ preputial/rectal smear

Swab Sample

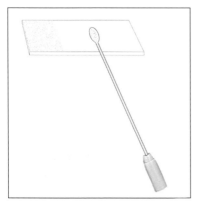

Fig 2.52 Roll the swab sample onto a microscope slide

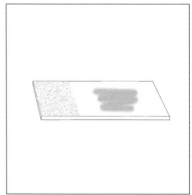

Fig 2.53 Dry

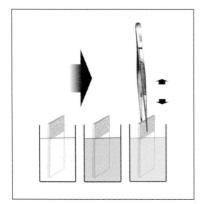

Fig 2.54 Fixate and stain

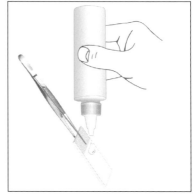

Fig 2.55 Rinse

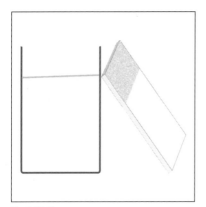

Fig 2.56 Dry

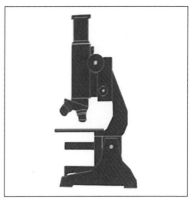

Fig 2.57 Microscopic examination

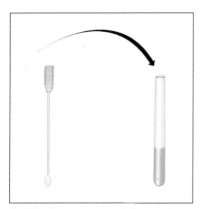

Fig 2.58 Transfer the sample into a culture tube (bacteriology)

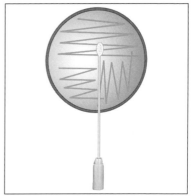

Fig 2.59 Smear the swab onto a fungal culture medium (mycology)

Cytology

- **Technique**

    - Make a smear
    - Roll the smear onto a microscope slide
    - Dry the smear
    - Fixate and stain the smear
    - Rinse the smear with water/distilled water
    - Dry the smear in a tilted position
    - Perform a microscopic examination

Bacteriology

- **Technique**

    - Transfer the swab sample into a culture tube
    - Dispatch the sample

Mycology

- **Technique**

    - Smear the swab sample onto a fungal culture medium

Skin Scrape

Indication

- Cytological/ectoparasitical/mycological skin examination

Skin Scrape: Examination for Ectoparasites (especially Demodex sp.)

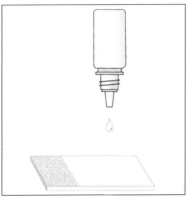

Fig 2.60 Apply a drop of paraffin

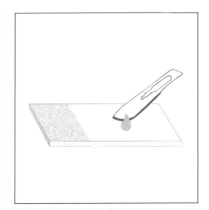

Fig 2.61 Add the sample

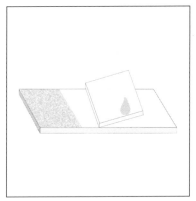

Fig 2.62 Place cover slide on top

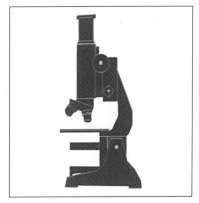

Fig 2.63 Microscopic examination

Skin Scrape: Cytological Examination

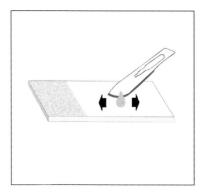

Fig 2.64 Apply and spread out the sample

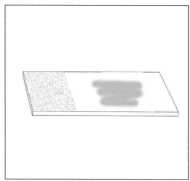

Fig 2.65 Dry

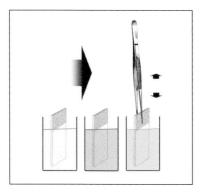

Fig 2.66 Fixate and stain

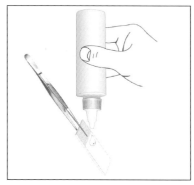

Fig 2.67 Rinse

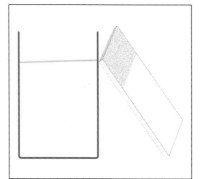

Fig 2.68 Dry

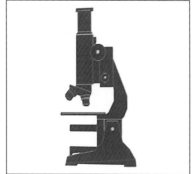

Fig 2.69 Microscopic examination

Parasitology

- **Technique**
  - Apply a drop of paraffin onto a microscope slide
  - Apply the sample onto the microscope slide
  - Place a cover slide on top
  - Perform a microscopic examination

Cytology

- **Technique**
  - Apply and spread out the sample onto a microscope slide
  - Dry the sample
  - Fixate and stain the sample
  - Rinse the sample with water/distilled water
  - Dry the sample in a tilted position
  - Perform a microscopic examination

Impression Smear/Skin Scrape

Indication

- Ulcerating Tumours, Eczema

Impression Smear

Fig 2.70 Apply the sample directly onto a microscope slide

Fig 2.71 Dry

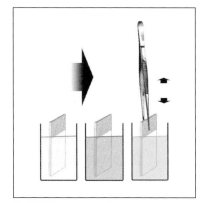

Fig 2.72 Fixate and stain

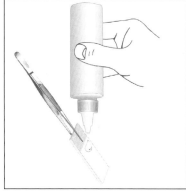

Fig 2.73 Rinse

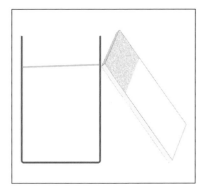

Fig 2.74 Dry

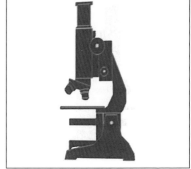

Fig 2.75 Microscopic examination

Cytology

- **Technique**
  - Dab/spread the sample directly onto a microscope slide
  - Dry the sample
  - Fixate and stain the sample
  - Rinse the sample with water/distilled water
  - Dry the sample in a tilted position
  - Perform a microscopic examination

Sticky Tape Impression

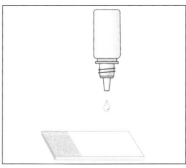

Fig 2.76 Apply one drop of paraffin onto a microscope slide

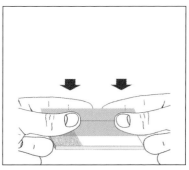

Fig 2.77 Apply some sticky tape onto a microscope slide

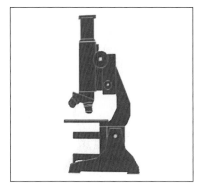

Fig 2.78 Microscopic examination

Sticky Tape Impression

• **Technique**
  - Apply one drop of paraffin onto a microscope slide
  - Dab the skin with some sticky tape
  - Apply the sticky tape onto a microscope slide
  - Perform a microscopic examination

Hair Sample

Indication

- Alopecia, hair breakage
- Dermatophytosis

Hair Sample: Examination of the Hair

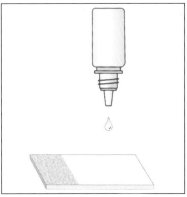

Fig 2.79 Apply one drop of paraffin to a microscope slide

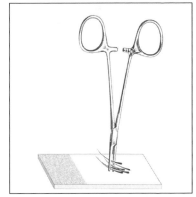

Fig 2.80 Add the hair sample

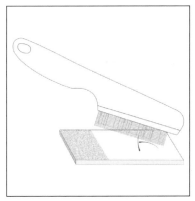

Fig 2.81 Apply the hair sample from the flea comb

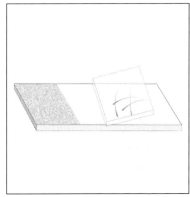

Fig 2.82 Add a cover slide

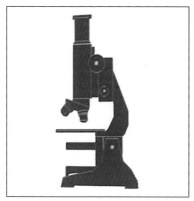

Fig 2.83 Microscopic examination

Hair Sample: Fungal Culture

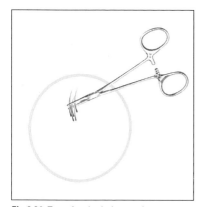

Fig 2.84 Transfer the hair sample onto a fungal culture medium

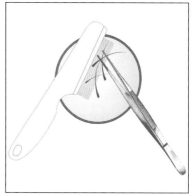

Fig 2.85 Transfer the hair sample onto a fungal culture medium

Hair Examination

- **Technique**
  - Apply one drop of paraffin onto a microscope slide
  - Transfer the hair sample onto a microscope slide
  - Apply a cover slide
  - Perform a microscopic examination

Mycology

- **Technique**
  - Transfer the hair sample onto a fungal culture medium

Urine Sample

Indication

- Urine chemistry, cytological and microbiological examination

Urine Sample: Urine Chemistry

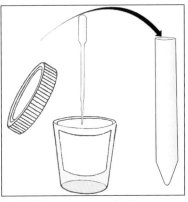

Fig 2.86 Transfer the sample into a centrifugation tube

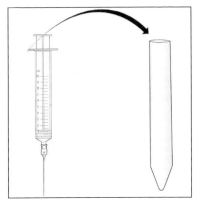

Fig 2.87 Transfer the sample into a centrifugation tube

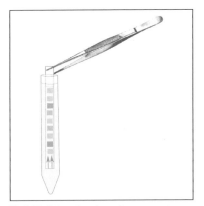

Fig 2.88 Urine chemistry via a test strip

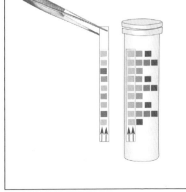

Fig 2.89 Analysis of the test strip

Urine Examination: Refractometry

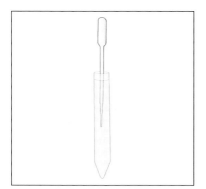

Fig 2.90 Take a sample for refractometry

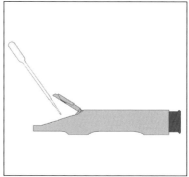

Fig 2.91 Apply the sample onto the refractometer

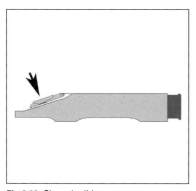

Fig 2.92 Close the lid

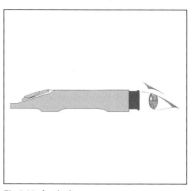

Fig 2.93 Analysis

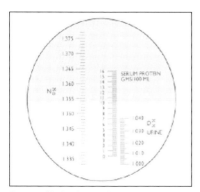

Fig 2.94 Evaluation scale

Urine Examination: Bacteriological Culture and Examination of the Sediment

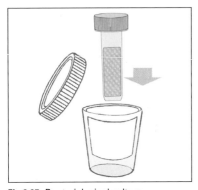

Fig 2.95 Bacteriological culture

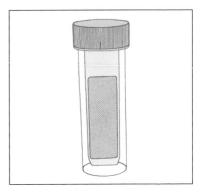

Fig 2.96 Bacteriological culture

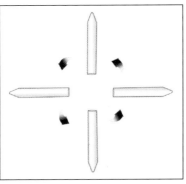

Fig 2.97 Centrifugation

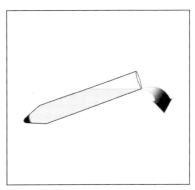

Fig 2.98 Decant the supernatant

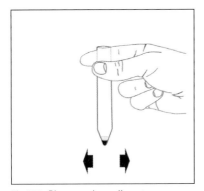

Fig 2.99 Plump up the sediment

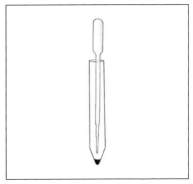

Fig 2.100 Pipette the sediment off

Urine Examination: Examination of the Sediment

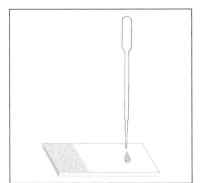

Fig 2.101 Apply the sample onto a microscope slide

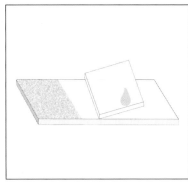

Fig 2.102 Apply a cover slide

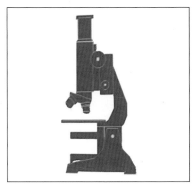

Fig 2.103 Microscopic examination (crystals)

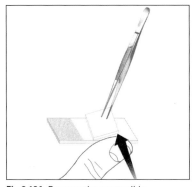

Fig 2.104 Remove the cover slide

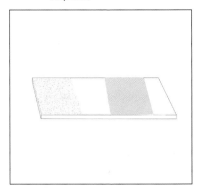

Fig 2.105 Dry

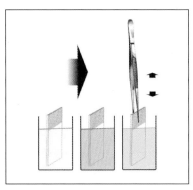

Fig 2.106 Fixate and stain

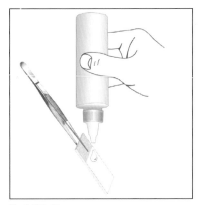

Fig 2.107 Rinse

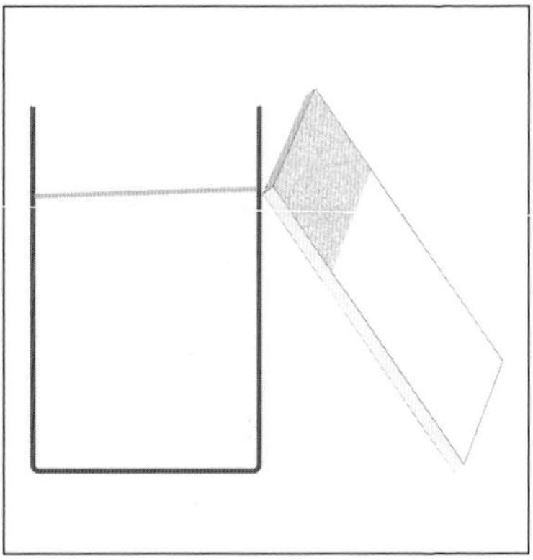

Fig 2.108 Dry

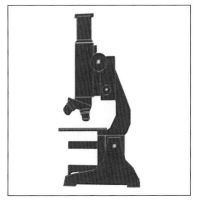

Fig 2.109 Microscopic examination

Urine Chemistry

- **Technique**

    - Transfer the urine sample into a pointed centrifugation tube
    - Dip the test strip into the tube
    - Analyse the results immediately with the colour scale on packaging

Refractometry

- **Technique**

    - Clean the refractometer and calibrate
    - Open the lid and apply one drop of urine
    - Close the lid and evaluate the specific gravity

Bacteriology

- **Technique**

    - Dip urine into the bacterial culture (Uricult®)
    - Close the tube

Cytology

- **Technique**

    - Centrifugation of the urine sample (c. 10 min at 3,000 rpm)
    - Decant the supernatant
    - Plump up the sediment
    - Transfer the sample onto a microscope slide
    - Add a cover slide
    - Perform a microscopic examination (crystals)
    - Remove the cover slide
    - Dry the sample
    - Fixate and stain the sample
    - Rinse the sample with water/distilled water
    - Dry the sample in a tilted position
    - Perform a microscopic examination (cytology)

Faecal Sample

Indication

• Parasitological and bacteriological examination

Coprological Examination: Flotation

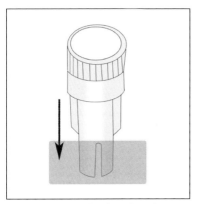

Fig 2.110 Press the fecalyser into the faeces

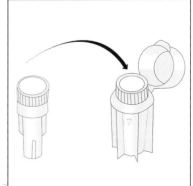

Fig 2.111 Transfer the fecalyser into a container

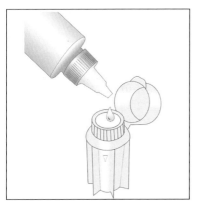

Fig 2.112 Add flotation fluid

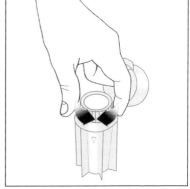

Fig 2.113 Twist the inset container several times

Faecal Sample: Flotation and Bacteriological Examination

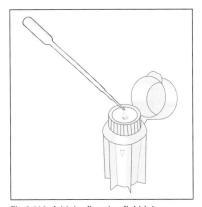

Fig 2.114 Add the flotation fluid (above meniscus)

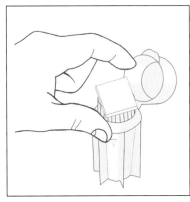

Fig 2.115 Apply a cover slide

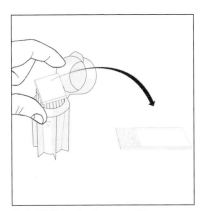

Fig 2.116 Transfer the cover slide to a microscope slide after 15 mins

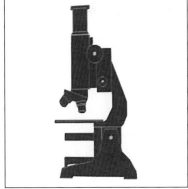

Fig 2.117 Microscopic examination

Faecal Sample: Plain Sample Preparation

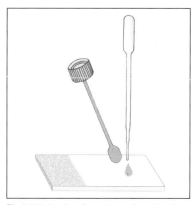

Fig 2.118 Apply a faecal sample and saline solution onto a microscope slide

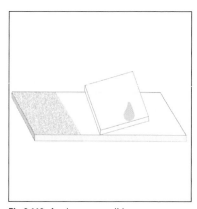

Fig 2.119 Apply a cover slide

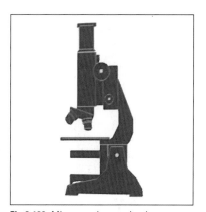

Fig 2.120 Microscopic examination

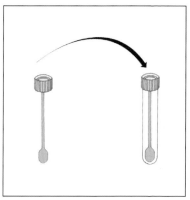

Fig 2.121 Dispatch of the sample possible in a transport container

Coprological Examination

Flotation

- **Technique**
  - Press the fecalyser into the faecal sample
  - Transfer the fecalyser into its container
  - Add the flotation fluid
  - Twist the inset container several times for mixing
  - Top up the flotation fluid with a pipette above the meniscus
  - Apply a cover slide
  - Wait c. 15 min
  - Transfer the cover slide onto a microscope slide
  - Perform a microscopic examination (oocyst)

Plain Sample Preparation

- **Technique**
  - Apply a rice grain sized faecal sample onto a microscope slide
  - Mix in two drops of saline
  - Apply a cover slide
  - Perform a microscopic examination (coccidia + oocyst)

Dispatch of the Sample

- **Technique**
  - Bacteriology
  - Protozoology (*Giardia* spp.)
  - Digestive products
  - Digestive enzymes

3 Cardiological Examination Methods

Case History

Principal Symptoms

- Performance insufficiency
- Respiratory distress
- Cough
- Syncope
- Nocturnal unrest
- Weight loss
- Paraparesis (especially cat)
- Cyanosis

Inspection

Indication

- Part of the general examination

Method

- **Technique**
    - Observation of the body position/stance and respiration at rest
    - Observation of the oral and preputial/vulval mucous membranes, neck including jugular veins, thorax and abdomen on the examination table (often in combination with palpation)

- **Evaluation criteria**
    - Size, shape, symmetry, respiratory rhythm (inspiration / expiration), jugular venous pulse, mucous membrane colour

Findings

- **Physiological**
  - Costoabdominal respiration/respiration rate 10–30/min
  - Mucous membrane colour: pink
  - No visible jugular venous pulse
- **Pathological**

  Respiration
  - Abdominal respiration (thoracic disease)
  - Costal respiration (abdominal disease)
  - Bradypnoea (sedation, CNS disease)
  - Tachypnoea (agitation, pain, systemic disease)
  - Inspiratory dyspnoea (upper airway disease)
  - Expiratory dyspnoea (lower airway disease)
  - Orthopnoea (lower airway disease)
  - Open-mouth breathing (lower airway disease)
  - Cheyne-Stokes breathing (CNS/cardiac disease, endocrine disease)

  Mucous membrane colour
  - Pallor (circulatory collapse/shock, anaemia)
  - Cyanosis (peripheral) (generalised blue colour of the mucous membranes as a result of heart failure and reduced cardiac output)
  - Cyanosis (central) (blue colour of the mucous membranes in the caudal body parts (vagina/prepuce) as a result of congenital heart disease with right to left shunt (Tetralogy of Fallot, Eisenmenger's syndrome – pulmonary hypertension with shunt reversal with persistent ductus arteriosus, ventricular septal-/atrial septal defect)
  - Cyanosis (paws/claws/pads of the hind limb) (aortic thromboembolism as a result of heart failure)

  Increased abdominal girth
  - Ascites/hepatomegaly (right-sided heart failure)

  State of nutrition
  - Cachexia (e.g., with left-sided heart failure)
  - Obesity (e.g., with right-sided heart failure)

  Congestion of jugular vein
  - Right-sided heart failure, pericardial effusion/cardiac tamponade
  - Jugular venous pulse
  - Tricuspid valve insufficiency, pulmonary valve stenosis, AV-dissociation as a result of right atrial contraction with closed tricuspid valve

Palpation

Indication

- Part of the general examination

Palpation

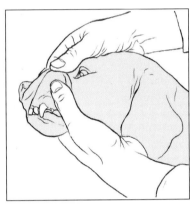

Fig 3.1 Measure the capillary refill time

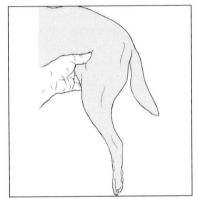

Fig 3.2 Compare the femoral arterial pulses

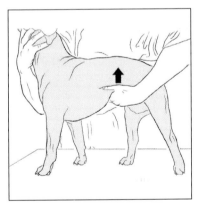

Fig 3.3 Hepatojugulary reflex

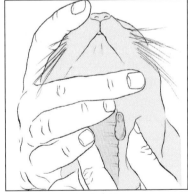

Fig 3.4 Palpate the thyroid

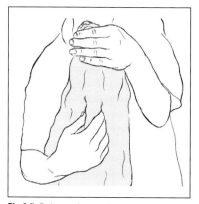

Fig 3.5 Palpate the trachea

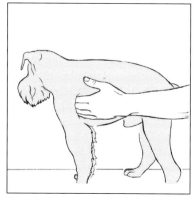

Fig 3.6 Palpate the cardiac apex beat

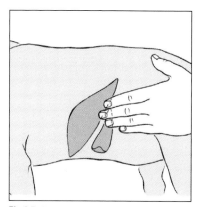

Fig 3.7 Palpate the liver and spleen

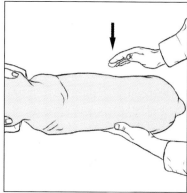

Fig 3.8 Fluid thrill

Method

- **Technique**

    Capillary refill time
    - Apply digital pressure to an area of unpigmented mucous membrane in the mouth
    - Let go and measure the time until the original mucous membrane colour has been reinstated

    Pulse
    - Feel the femoral arterial pulse wave with flatly placed fingertips of the index and middle finger
    - Palpate and compare both femoral arterial pulses with the heart rate via auscultation
    - Evaluate the frequency, regularity, evenness, quality (size and strength) and arterial filling/tension

    Hepatojugulary reflex
    - Lift the cranial abdomen while looking at both jugular veins
    - Evaluate jugular congestion, dilation and venous pulse

    Thyroid
    - Palpate and compare both sides of the ventral neck region with index/middle finger

    Trachea
    - Feel the trachea between your thumb and index/middle finger
    - Compress the trachea slightly

    Cardiac apex beat
    - Place the palms of your hands on both sides of the cranial thorax

    Liver/spleen
    - Feel the organ edges (possibly while the patient is standing)

    Abdomen (fluid thrill)
    - Tap the lateral abdominal wall with the fingers of one hand, while the other hand is flatly placed against the collateral side feeling a pressure wave (in case of abdominal effusion)

Findings

- **Physiological**

  Capillary refill time
  - < 2 sec

  Pulse
  - Regular, even, of medium size, strength, arterial filling and tension, no pulse deficits

  Hepatojugulary reflex
  - No evidence of jugular vein congestion/-dilation

  Thyroid
  - Not palpable

  Trachea
  - Unable to elicit a coughing reflex with moderate tracheal compression

  Cardiac apex beat
  - Apex beat on the left cranial thoracic wall
  - Hypokinetic: physiological with a broad thorax/obesity

  Liver/spleen
  - Caudal liver edges are hardly palpable

  Abdomen (fluid thrill)
  - No fluid pressure wave palpable

- **Pathological**

  Capillary refill time
  - > 2 sec (reduced cardiac output/peripheral impairment of blood supply)

  Pulse: hyperkinetic
  - Pulsus celer (fast), altus (high amplitude) et durus (hard) (aortic insufficiency, anaemia, hyperthyroidism, fever, persistent ductus arteriosus)
  - Pulsus celer (fast) et parvus (small amplitude) (Hypovolaemia)

  Pulse: hypokinetic
  - Pulsus tardus (slow), parvus (small amplitude) et mollis (soft) (aortic stenosis, pulmonary stenosis, shock)
  - Pulsus alternans (variable strength) (heart failure)

- Pulsus paradoxus (reduced strength in inspiration) (pericardial effusion/cardiac tamponade)
- Pulse deficit (difference between the heart and pulse rate) (haemodynamically ineffective extrasystoles, absolute tachyarrhythmia)
- Missing pulse with a physiological heart rate (vessel occluding disease process)

Hepatojugular reflex
- Congestion/dilation of the jugular vein (right-sided heart failure)

Thyroid
- Goitre (hyperthyroidism, abscess, tumour)

Trachea
- Cough (tracheitis/tracheobronchitis)

Cardiac apex beat
- Hyperkinetic: hyperthyroidism, aortic insufficiency, anaemia
- Hypokinetic: shock, pericardial effusion/cardiac tamponade, pulmonary emphysema, pneumothorax
- Changed position (cardiomegaly)

Liver/spleen
- Increased liver size (e.g., right-sided heart failure, tumour)

Abdomen (fluid thrill)
- Positive (abdominal effusion)

Auscultation

Indication

- Part of the general examination

Auscultation

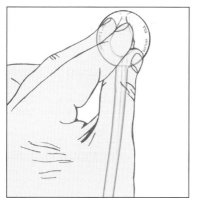

Fig 3.9 Auscultation with a stethoscope

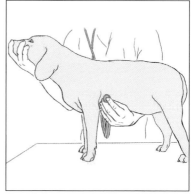

Fig 3.10 Auscultation while occluding the nostrils

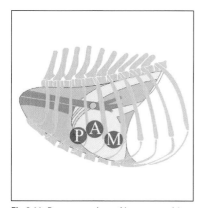

Fig 3.11 Puncta maxima of heart sounds (left): P = pulmonary valve; A = aortic valve; M = mitral valve

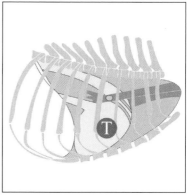

Fig 3.12 Puncta maxima of heart sounds (right): T = tricuspid valve

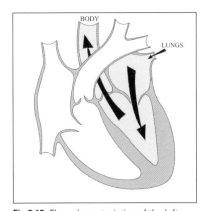

Fig 3.13 Flow characteristics of the left heart (Korper = body; Lunge = lung)

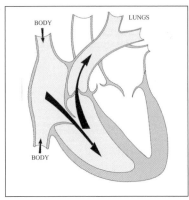

Fig 3.14 Flow characteristics of the right heart

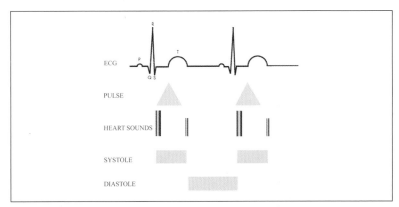

Fig 3.15 Heart cycle (ECG, pulse, heart sounds, systole, diastole)

Method

- **Technique**

  - Auscultation between the third and fifth intercostal space of the left, right and cranial thoracic wall
  - Auscultation while the patient is standing
  - Perform a comparing palpation of the femoral arterial pulse
  - Provide a calm environment, best done with closed eyes, consider occluding the nostrils momentarily
  - Consider distracting purring cats by having a water tap running

- **Heart sounds**

  - Evaluate the number of sounds (usually two), heart rate, separation/division, regularity, evenness, quality (loud, quiet, drumming) and clicks

- **Heart murmurs**

  Time of occurrence
  - Systole (holosystolic, mesosystolic, late systolic)
  - Diastole (early diastolic, mesodiastolic, presystolic)
  - Continuous (systolic/diastolic, machine-like)

  Volume
  - Grade 1 very quiet (audible only during apnoea)
  - Grade 2 quiet (audible after a brief period of time)
  - Grade 3 medium-loud (immediately audible)
  - Grade 4 loud
  - Grade 5 very loud (audible while the stethoscope is lifted off the thoracic wall)

  Puncta maxima
  - Pulmonary valve: left thoracic wall, third intercostal space below the costochondral junction
  - Aortic valve: left thoracic wall, fourth intercostal space above the costochondral junction
  - Mitral valve: left thoracic wall, fifth intercostal space at the costochondral junction
  - Tricuspid valve: right thoracic wall, fourth intercostal space at the costochondral junction

Sound character
- Crescendo (rising sound)
- Decrescendo (subsiding sound)
- Crescendo – decrescendo
- Sound conduction
- Extracardial (respiratory, peristaltic, pericardial or rubbing sounds)

- **Heart cycle**

Flow characteristics
- Left heart: lung → pulmonary veins → atrium → mitral valve → ventricle → aortic valve → aorta → body
- Right heart: body → V. cava → atrium → tricuspid valve → ventricle → pulmonary valve → pulmonary artery → lung

Pulse
- Haemodynamic pressure wave during systole

Heart sounds
- 1. Heart sound – closure of the mitral and tricuspid (atrioventricular) valves
- 2. Heart sound – closure of the aortic and pulmonary (semilunar) valves
- Systole – ventricular expulsion phase
- Diastole – ventricular filling phase

Findings During Auscultation

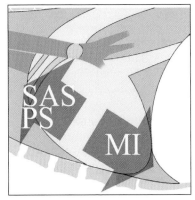

Fig 3.16 Conduction of heart sounds (left)

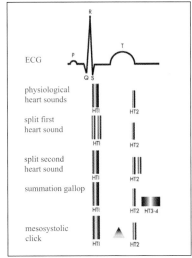

Fig 3.18
Pathological heart sounds (ECG –
physiological heart sounds – split first heart
sound – split second heart sound-
summation gallop – mesosystolic click)

Fig 3.19 *(below)*
Heart murmurs (holosystolic band shaped –
mesosystolic spindle shaped – early
diastolic subsiding – continuous (machine
sound) – AV-valve insufficiency –
semilunar valve stenosis – persistent
ductus arteriosus

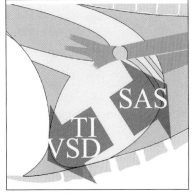

Fig 3.17 Conduction of heart sounds (right)

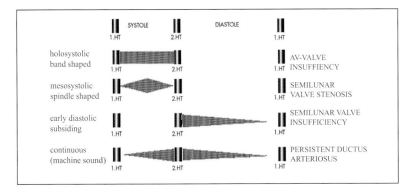

Findings

- **Physiological**

  Heart rate
  - Dog (70–160/min)
  - Cat (160–220/min)
  - Puppies (> 220/min)

  Heart rhythm
  - Regular/even heart rhythm

  Heart sounds
  - Regular/even, well separated heart sounds
  - Split first heart sound (physiological in large dog breeds)
  - Split second heart sound (physiologically respiration dependent)

- **Pathological**

  Heart rate
  - Tachycardia: dog (> 180/min.); cat (> 220/min.); puppies (> 220/min.)
  - Bradycardia: dog (< 60/min.); cat (< 100/min)

  Heart rhythm
  - Tachycardic arrhythmias
  - Bradycardic arrhythmias

  Heart sounds
  - Split first heart sound (ventricular extrasystole)
  - Split second heart sound (pulmonary valve stenosis, atrial septal defect, right bundle branch block, dirofilariosis)
  - Summation gallop (heart failure)
  - Systolic click (mitral valve prolapse)

Heart murmurs

Systolic
  - Holosystolic/band shaped (mitral valve insufficiency)
  - Holosystolic/band shaped (tricuspid valve insufficiency)
  - Mesosystolic/spindle shaped (sub aortic stenosis)
  - Mesosystolic/spindle shaped (pulmonary valve stenosis)
  - Holosystolic/band shaped (ventricular septal defect)

Diastolic
  - ([Sub]aortic insufficiency) (early diastolic/subsiding)
  - Early diastolic/subsiding (pulmonary valve insufficiency)

Continuous
  - Machine sound (persistent ductus arteriosus)

Conduction of heart murmurs

Towards cranial
  - Sub aortic stenosis (SAS)
  - Pulmonary valve stenosis (PS)
  - Persistent ductus arteriosus (PDA)

Towards caudal
  - Mitral valve insufficiency (MI)
  - Tricuspid valve insufficiency (TI)
  - Ventricular septal defect (VSD)

X-Ray Study

Indication

- Heart/respiratory disease

X-Ray Study

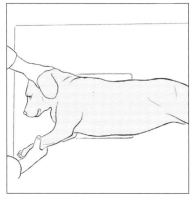

Fig 3.20 Patient positioning (lateral view)

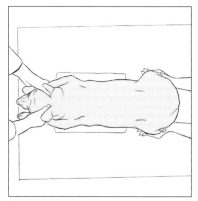

Fig 3.21 Patient positioning (dorsoventral view)

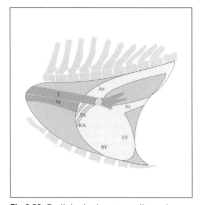

Fig 3.22 Radiological anatomy (lateral projection)

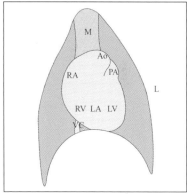

Fig 3.23 Radiological anatomy (dorsoventral projection)

Measuring the Heart Size

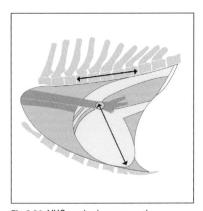

Fig 3.24 VHS method: measure the longitudinal axis

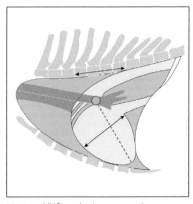

Fig 3.25 VHS method: measure the horizontal axis

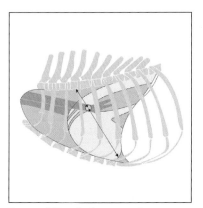

Fig 3.26 ICR method: measure the horizontal axis

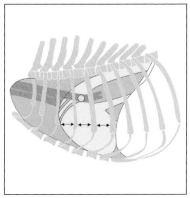

Fig 3.27 ICR method: measure the horizontal axis

Method

- **Technique**
  - Perform risk/benefit assessment (if the patient is dyspnoeic)
  - Plan and agree the proposed procedure with colleagues and owners
  - Fully inform the owner (consider questions about pregnancy and age range)
  - Handle the patient calmly and in a coordinated manner
  - Possible distraction
  - Projection of two views if at all possible
  - Thoracic radiographs generally in maximum inspiration (check X-ray for elevation of diaphragm)
  - Left and right lateral views
  - Second X-ray view usually in sternal/prone position (dorsoventral)
  - Opposing ribs should overlap perfectly

- **Radiological anatomy**
  - Right atrium (RA)
  - Left atrium (LA)
  - Right ventricle (RV)
  - Left ventricle (LV)
  - Pulmonary trunk/truncus pulmonalis (TP)
  - Left pulmonary artery (LPA)
  - Right pulmonary artery (RPA)
  - Aorta (Ao)
  - Vena cava (Vc)
  - Mediastinum (M)
  - Trachea (T)

- **Measure the heart size**
  - VHS-Method (vertebral heart size)
  - Measure the longitudinal axis (bifurcation to apex), compare this with the sum of the vertebral lengths from T4
  - Measure the horizontal axis (maximum cardiac width 90° to the longitudinal axis)
  - Compare this with the sum of the vertebral lengths from T4
  - VHS = vertebral lengths of the longitudinal axis + vertebral lengths of the horizontal axis (normal range in the dog: 8.5–10.5)
  - ICR method (intercostal room)
  - Measure the longitudinal axis of the thoracic cavity (thoracic vertebrae-bifurcation-sternum), normal value in the dog: cardiac height should be two-thirds of the thoracic cavity
  - Measure the horizontal axis (maximum cardiac width) by counting the intercostal spaces (normal range in the dog: heart width 2.5–3.5 intercostal spaces or 50–60 per cent of the thoracic diameter)

X-Ray Findings

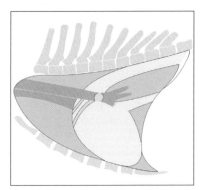

Fig 3.28 Physiological heart size (lateral)

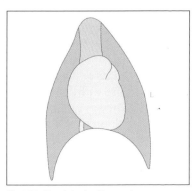

Fig 3.29 Physiological heart size (dorsoventral)

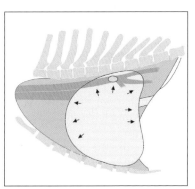

Fig 3.30 Bilateral atrial enlargement (l)

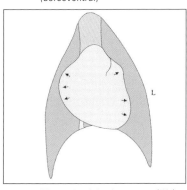

Fig 3.31 Bilateral atrial enlargement (d/v)

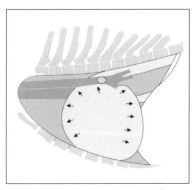

Fig 3.32 Generalised cardiomegaly (l)

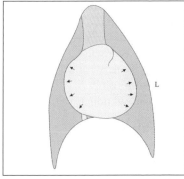

Fig 3.33 Generalised cardiomegaly (d/v)

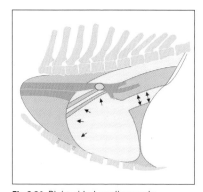

Fig 3.34 Right-sided cardiomegaly (RA+RV) (l)

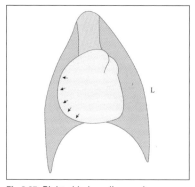

Fig 3.35 Right-sided cardiomegaly (RA+RV) (d/v)

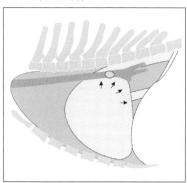

Fig 3.36 Left-sided cardiomegaly (LA+LV) (l)

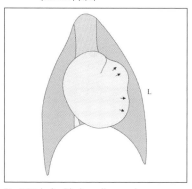

Fig 3.37 Left-sided cardiomegaly (LA+LV) (d/v)

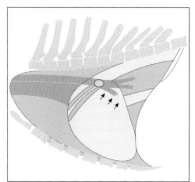

Fig 3.38 Left-sided atrial enlargement (LA) (l)

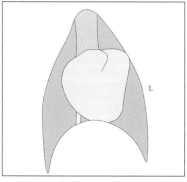

Fig 3.39 Left-sided atrial enlargement (LA) (d/v)

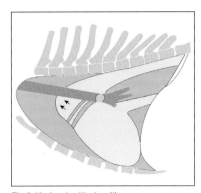

Fig 3.40 Aortic dilation (l)

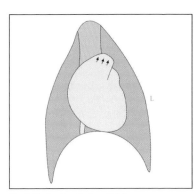

Fig 3.41 Aortic dilation (d/v)

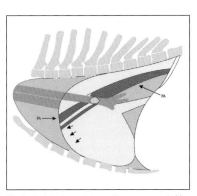

Fig 3.42 Dilation of the pulmonary trunk (l)

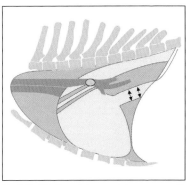

Fig 3.43 Dilation of the caudal vena cava (l)

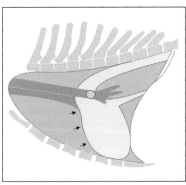

Fig 3.44 Microcardia (l)

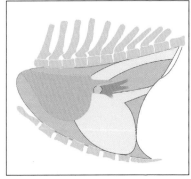

Fig 3.45 Persistent right fourth aortic arc

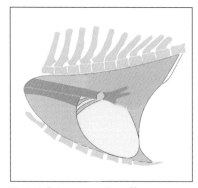

Fig 3.46 Pulmonary oedema (I)

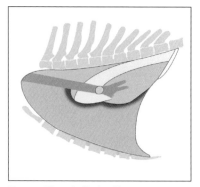

Fig 3.47 Pleural effusion (I)

Findings

- **Physiological**
  - Nothing abnormal to detect (NAD)

- **Pathological**

  Heart size

  Bilateral atrial enlargement
  - Chronic AV-valve insufficiency (mitral valve/tricuspid valve)
  - Ventricular septal defect (VSD)
  - Dilated cardiomyopathy (DCMP)

  Generalised cardiomegaly
  - Pericardial effusion/cardiac tamponade

  Right-sided cardiomegaly (RA + RV)
  - Cor pulmonale (as a result of respiratory disease)
  - Pulmonary valve stenosis (PS)
  - Tricuspid valve insufficiency (TI)
  - Atrial septal defect (ASD)
  - Tetralogy of Fallot
  - Shunt-reversal (Eisenmenger Syndrome)
  - Persistent ductus arteriosus (PDA)
  - Atrial/ventricular septal defect (ASD/VSD)

  Left-sided cardiomegaly (LA + LV)
  - Cardiomyopathy
  - Mitral valve insufficiency (MI)
  - (Sub-)aortic stenosis and aortic insufficiency (SAS/AI)
  - Ventricular septal defect (VSD)
  - Persistent ductus arteriosus (PDA)

Left atrial enlargement (LA)
- Mitral valve insufficiency (MI)
- Persistent ductus arteriosus (PDA)
- Hypertrophic cardiomyopathy (HCMP)

Aortic dilation
- (Sub-)aortic stenosis (SAS) with post stenotic dilation
- Persistent ductus arteriosus (PDA)
- Persistent right fourth aortic arch
- Arterial hypertension (especially hyperthyroidism in cats)

Dilation of the pulmonary trunk
- Persistent ductus arteriosus (PDA)
- Ventricular septal defect (VSD)
- Congestive heart failure (dilation of the pulmonary veins)
- Dirofilariosis (dilation of the pulmonary arteries)
- Pulmonary valve stenosis (PS) (dilation of the pulmonary trunk)

Reduction in size of the pulmonary vessels
- Tetralogy of Fallot (pulmonary veins)
- Pulmonary valve stenosis (PS) (pulmonary veins)
- Hypovolaemia

Dilation of the caudal vena cava
- Right-sided heart failure (tricuspid valve insufficiency)
- Pericardial effusion/ cardiac tamponade

Heart shape
- Rounded cardiac silhouette (pericardial effusion)
- Valentine heart (d/v) (hypertrophic cardiomyopathy)
- Reversed D shape (right sided enlargement)

Heart position
- Shifting of the axis to the right (right cardiac enlargement)
- Shifting of the axis to the left (left cardiac enlargement)

Thorax
- Pleural effusion
- Heart base tumour

Abdomen
- Ascites (right-sided heart failure)
- Hepato-/splenomegaly (right-sided heart failure)

Trachea
- Elevation of the trachea (cardiac enlargement)
- Tracheal collapse (right sided overload)

Lung
- Cardiac pulmonary oedema (left-sided heart failure)
- Pneumonia (right cardiac overload)

Oesophagus
- Megaoesophagus (e.g., right-sided persistent fourth aortic arch)

Electrocardiography (ECG)

Indication

- Cardiac arrhythmias
- Anaesthetic/intensive care monitoring

ECG

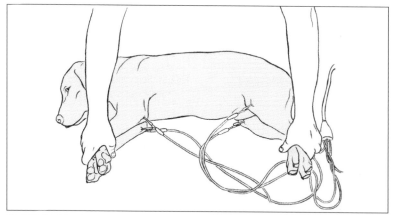

Fig 3.48 Limb leads

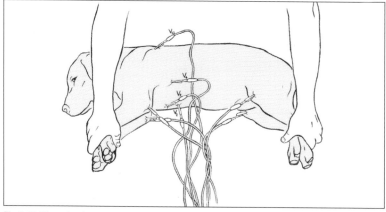

Fig 3.49 Chest leads

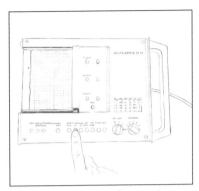

Fig 3.50 Select the recording speed

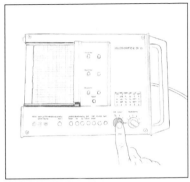

Fig 3.51 Select the recording amplitude

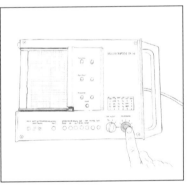

Fig 3.52 Select the leads (1–6)

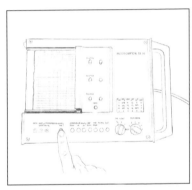

Fig 3.53 Press start

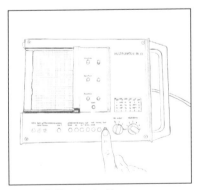

Fig 3.54 Calibration 1 mV

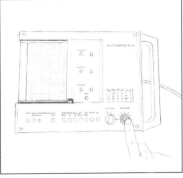

Fig 3.55 Switch recording lead

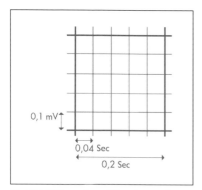

Fig 3.56 ECG readings (50mm/sec and 1cm = 1mV)

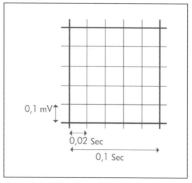

Fig 3.57 ECG readings (25mm/sec and 1cm = 1mV)

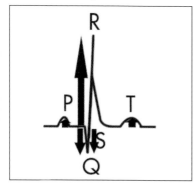

Fig 3.58 Amplitude formation of a normal P-QRS-T complex

	Dog (mV)	Cat (mV)
P	< 0,4	< 0,2
Q	< 0,5	< 0,5
R	< 2,5 (< 25 kg BW) < 3,0 (> 25kg BW)	< 0,9
S	< 0,35 (< 25% vonR)	

Fig 3.59 Amplitude readings (normal values)

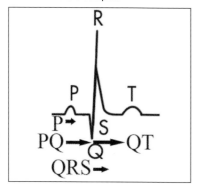

Fig 3.60 Time/interval readings

	Dog (sec)	Cat (sec)
P	< 0,04	< 0,04
PQ	< 0,13	< 0,09
QRS	< 0,05	< 0,04
QT	< 0,25	< 0,18

Fig 3.61 Time/interval readings (normal values)

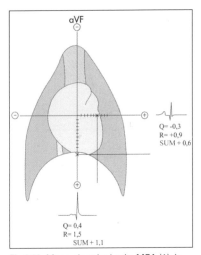

Fig 3.62 Mean electrical axis, MEA (1), in illustration: sum

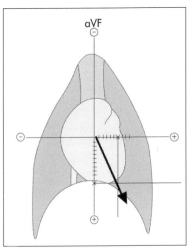

Fig 3.63 Mean electrical axis (2)

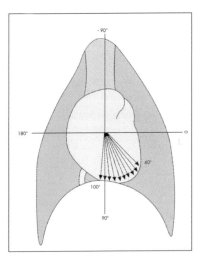

Fig 3.64 Physiological mean electrical axis (dog)

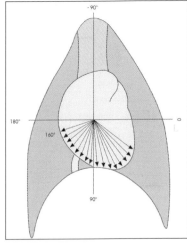

Fig 3.65 Physiological mean electrical axis (cat)

Method

- **Technique**
    - Placement of the electrodes
    - Patient in lateral recumbency (standing if in respiratory distress)
    - Stretch the crocodile clips (they are quite painful, consider filing the teeth down!)
    - Place the crocodile clip electrodes onto a skin fold
    - Moisten the skin/electrodes with spirit/electrode gel)
    - Position of electrodes (standard leads)
        - Red (right forelimb proximal of the olecranon)
        - Yellow (left forelimb proximal of the olecranon)
        - Green (left hind limb knee fold)
        - Black (usually right hind limb knee fold)
    - Position of electrodes (chest leads)
        - White rV2 (CV5RL): right chest wall, fifth intercostal space, parasternal
        - White V2 (CV6LL): left chest wall, sixth intercostal space, parasternal
        - White V4 (CV6LU): left chest wall, sixth costochondral junction
        - White V10: between shoulder blades at level with Th6–7

- **Device operation**
    - Example type Multiscriptor EK 33® Hellige[HJ1]
    - Select the paper speed 25mm/sec, 50mm/sec
    - Select the recording amplitude, usually 1cm/mV (¼cm/mV, ½cm/mV, 2cm/mV)
    - Select the leads (program 1–6)
        - Program 1 (leads I, II, III)
        - Program 2 (leads aVR, aVL, aVF)
        - Program 3 (leads V1, V2, V3)
        - Program 4 (leads V4, V5, V6)
    - Press the start button
    - Calibration button (calibration 1cm)
    - Switch settings while writing. Fine tune the amplitude with filter button. Order of studies:
        - 1. Calibration
        - 2. Program 1 (I, II, III) at 25mm/sec, 1cm/mV
        - 3. Program 1 (I, II, III) at 50mm/sec, 1cm/mV
        - 4. Program 2 (I, II, III) at 50mm/sec, 1cm/mV

- **ECG measures**
  - Heart rate/min at 25mm/sec
    - Number of QRS-complexes in 6 sec (15cm) × 10 at 50mm/sec
    - Number of QRS-complexes in 6 sec (30cm) × 10
  - Amplitudes (lead II), P, Q, R, S, T at 1cm = 1mV: 1mm = 0.1mV
  - Time periods (lead II)
    - P, PQ, QRS, QT, RR
    - At 25mm/sec: 1mm = 0.04 sec
    - At 50mm/sec: 1mm = 0.02 sec
  - Mean electrical axis (vector-method)
    1. Measure and add up the net-QRS-amplitudes of leads I and aVF (or leads I and III).
       Example: Lead I: Q = –0.3mV   Lead aVF: Q = –0.4mV
                      R = +0.9mV   R = +1.5mV
                       + 0.6   +1.1
    2. Record the values in the appropriate axis
    3. Plot the intersection of the vertical and horizontal lines through these values
    4. Mean electrical heart axis = connecting line between the graph origin and the intersection found in step 3

- **Evaluation criteria**
  - Heart rhythm
  - Heart rate
  - Amplitudes
  - Time periods
  - Mean electrical axis

ECG – Findings

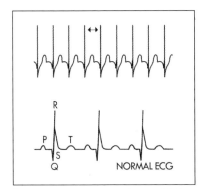

Fig 3.66 Sinus tachycardia (normal ECG)

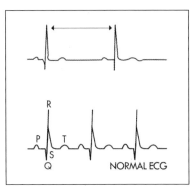

Fig 3.67 Sinus bradycardia (normal ECG)

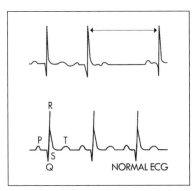

Fig 3.68 SA-Block/sinus arrest (normal ECG)

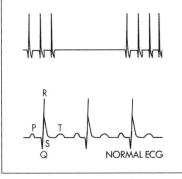

Fig 3.69 Sick-sinus-syndrome (normal ECG)

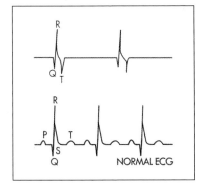

Fig 3.70 Atrial standstill (normal ECG)

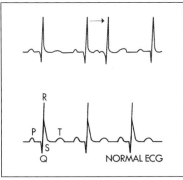

Fig 3.71 Supraventricular premature complex (normal ECG)

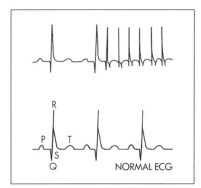

Fig 3.72 Supraventricular tachycardia

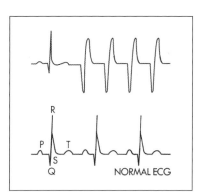

Fig 3.73 Atrial flutter/fibrillation

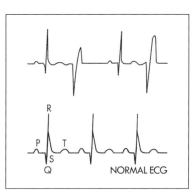

Fig 3.74 Ventricular ectopic complex

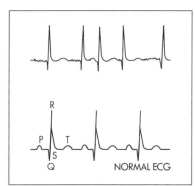

Fig 3.75 Ventricular tachycardia

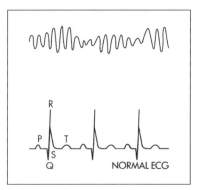

Fig 3.76 Ventricular fibrillation

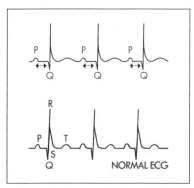

Fig 3.77 First degree AV-block

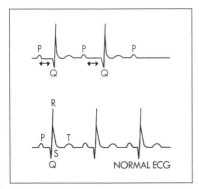

Fig 3.78 Second degree AV-block (Mobitz Type 1)

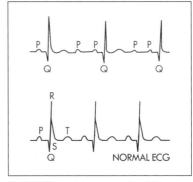

Fig 3.79 Second degree AV-block (Mobitz Type 2)

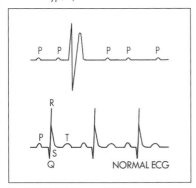

Fig 3.80 Third degree AV-block

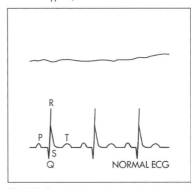

Fig 3.81 Asystole

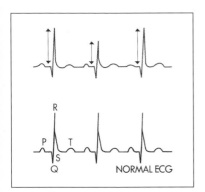

Fig 3.82 Electrical alternans

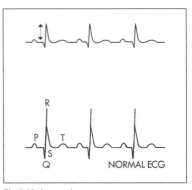

Fig 3.83 Low voltage

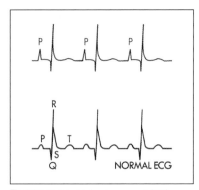

Fig 3.84 Right atrial enlargement (RA)

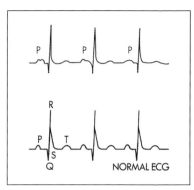

Fig 3.85 Left atrial enlargement (LA)

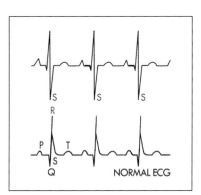

Fig 3.86 Right ventricular enlargement (RV)

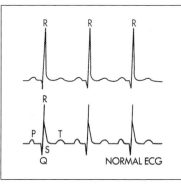

Fig 3.87 Left ventricular enlargement (LV)

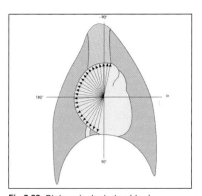

Fig 3.88 Right axis deviation (dog)

Pathological Findings

- **Sinus Tachycardia**

  ECG – findings
  - Heart rate > 180/min (dog), > 220/min (puppy/cat)

  Causes
  - Pain
  - Fever
  - Anaemia
  - Hyperthyroidism
  - Excitement/sympathetic tone
  - Heart failure

- **Sinus bradycardia**

  ECG – findings
  - Heart rate < 60/min (dog), < 100/min (cat)

  Causes
  - Parasympathetic tone/vagal tone
  - Carotid sinus irritation (collar)
  - Cerebral pressure
  - Hypothyroidism
  - Medication/anaesthetic agents (digoxin, xylazine)
  - Heart failure

- **SA-block/sinus arrest**

  ECG – findings
  - Rest between P-QRS-T-complexes (often longer than two normal RR-intervals)

  Causes
  - Parasympathetic tone/vagal tone
  - Sinus node dysfunction

- **Sick-sinus-syndrome**

  ECG – findings
  - Alternating sinus bradycardia/sinus arrest with paroxysmal supraventricular extrasystole/supraventricular tachycardia

Causes
- Sinus node dysfunction
- Genetic causes (Miniature Schnauzer)

- **Atrial standstill**

ECG – findings
- Reduced heart rate (escape rhythm)
- Missing P-wave
- Prolonged QRS-Interval
- Prolonged QT-Interval
- Reduced R-wave voltage
- Tall and spiked T-waves

Causes
- Hyperkalaemia

- **Supraventricular premature complex**

ECG – findings
- Premature P-wave
- Slightly distorted P-waves

Causes
- Vegetative dystonia
- Medication (e.g., digoxin, anaesthetic agents)
- AV-valve insufficiency

- **Atrial flutters/fibrillation**

ECG – findings
- Increased heart rate
- Irregular rhythm
- Missing P-waves

Causes
- Atrial myocardial disease (especially giant breeds)
- Drugs (e.g. digoxin)

- **Ventricular ectopic complex**

ECG – findings
- Premature, deformed QRS-complex
- P-waves unconnected to QRS-complex
- Complete compensatory pause (ventricular escape complex)
- Bigeminy: every second complex is premature
- Trigeminy: every third complex is premature

Causes
- Electrolyte imbalances
- Medications (e.g., digoxin, xylazine, barbiturates, antiarrhythmic drugs)
- Heart failure
- Metabolic acidosis
- Septicaemia/endotoxaemia
- Hypoxia

- **Ventricular tachycardia**

ECG – findings
- Ventricular premature complexes in rapid succession (three or more)
- Distorted QRS-complexes

Causes
- Electrolyte imbalances
- Medications(e.g., digoxin, phenobarbitone, antiarrhythmic drugs)
- Heart failure
- Metabolic acidosis
- Septicaemia/endotoxaemia
- Hypoxia

- **Ventricular fibrillation**

ECG – findings
- Undulations (fine/coarse) of the baseline
- QRS-complexes present?

Causes
- Electrolyte imbalances
- Medications (e.g., digoxin, phenobarbitone, antiarrhythmic drugs)
- Heart failure/hypoxia
- Metabolic acidosis
- Septicaemia/endotoxaemia

- **First grade AV-block**

ECG – findings
- Prolonged PQ-interval > 0.13 sec (dog), > 0.10 sec (cat)

Causes
- Physiological
- Parasympathetic tone/vagal tone
- Medications (digoxin, antiarrhythmic drugs)
- Hyperkalaemia
- AV-node-degeneration

- **Second degree AV-block (Mobitz Type 1)**

ECG – findings
- Irregular rhythm
- Normal P-waves
- Progressively prolonged PQ-Interval until absence of QRS-complex occurs (Wenckebach – Phenomenon)

Causes
- Parasympathetic tone/vagal tone
- Medications (e.g., digoxin, xylazine)
- Hyperkalaemia, hypocalcaemia
- AV-node degeneration
- Cardiomyopathy/myocarditis
- Aortic stenosis/ventricular septal defect

- **Second degree AV-block (Mobitz Type 2)**

ECG – findings
- Regular rhythm
- P-waves without subsequent QRS-complexes
- Conduction of only every second, third or fourth Impulse

Causes
- Parasympathetic tone/vagal tone
- Medications (e.g., digoxin, xylazine)
- Hyperkalaemia, hypocalcaemia
- AV-node degeneration
- Cardiomyopathy/myocarditis
- Aortic stenosis/ventricular septal defect

- **Third degree AV-block**

ECG – findings
- P-waves and QRS-complexes are unconnected (dissociation between atrial and ventricular activity)
- Slow ventricular escape rhythm
- Heart rate: < 50/min (dog), < 100/min (cat)

Causes
- Parasympathetic tone/vagal tone
- Medications (e.g., digoxin, xylazine)
- Hyperkalaemia, hypocalcaemia
- AV-node-degeneration
- Cardiomyopathy/myocarditis
- Aortic stenosis/ventricular septal defect

- **Asystole**

  ECG – findings
  - Baseline without any pulses (no measurable cardiac activity)

  Causes
  - Terminal heart disease
  - Hyperkalaemia
  - Metabolic acidosis
  - Third degree AV-block without escape rhythms

- **Electrical alternans**

  ECG – findings
  - Alternating variation in QRS amplitude

  Causes
  - Heart failure
  - Pericardial effusion/cardiac tamponade

- **Low voltage**

  ECG – findings
  - Decreased voltage of R-waves (< 1mV)

  Causes
  - Obesity
  - Pericardial effusion/cardiac tamponade

- **Right atrial (RA) enlargement**

  ECG – findings
  - Tall and spiky P-wave (P-pulmonale) amplitude: > 0.4mV (dog), > 0.2mV (cat)

- **Left atrial (LA) enlargement**

  ECG – findings
  - Prolonged and broad (sometimes notched) P-Wave (P-mitrale)
  - Interval: > 0.04mV (dog/cat)

- **Right ventricular (RV) enlargement**

  ECG – findings
  - S-waves present in leads I, II, III
  - Right axis deviation
  - Axis: 100° to −75° (dog), 160° to −75° (cat)
  - Deep S-waves in V3

- **Left ventricular (LV) enlargement**

  ECG – findings
  - Possibly tall R-waves amplitude: > 3.0 mV (dog), > 0.9 mV (cat)
  - Possibly prolonged QRS-complex: > 0.05 sec (dog)

- **Right axis deviation**

  ECG – findings
  - Shift of the mean electrical axis to right (right axis).
    Axis: 100° to −75° (dog), 160° to −75° (cat)

  Causes
  - Right ventricular enlargement

- **Hyperkalaemia**

  ECG – findings
  - Atrial standstill
  - Progressive bradycardia
  - Flat or missing P-wave
  - Prolonged PQ-interval
  - Prolonged QRS-interval
  - Shortened QT-interval ST-depression
  - Increased amplitude of T-wave, narrow and spiked

- **Hypokalaemia**

  ECG – findings
  - Tachycardia/tachyarrhythmia)
  - Prolonged QT-interval
  - ST-depression
  - Decreased and prolonged amplitude of T- wave, flat and broad

- **Hypercalcaemia**

  ECG – findings
  - Tachycardia (tachyarrhythmia)
  - Shortened QT-interval

- **Hypocalcaemia**

  ECG – findings
  - Tachycardia (tachyarrhythmia)
  - Prolonged QT–interval

- **Digoxin**

  ECG – findings
  - AV-block
  - Sinus bradycardia/sinus standstill
  - Ventricular ectopic complexes/ventricular tachycardia
  - Supraventricular premature complexes/supraventricular tachycardia/atrial fibrillation (in presence of bradycardia)

- **Xylazine**

  ECG – findings
  - Sinus bradycardia/sinus standstill
  - AV-block
  - Ventricular ectopic complexes

- **Lidocaine**

  ECG – findings
  - Sinus bradycardia/sinus standstill
  - AV-block

Complications

- Muscle tremors
- Electrical interactions
- Painful crocodile forceps

Ultrasound Examination

Indication

- Suspected acquired or congenital heart diseases
- Therapy monitoring

Positioning of the Patient

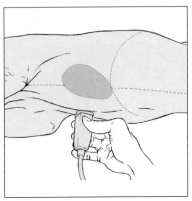

Fig 3.89 Examination in right lateral recumbency

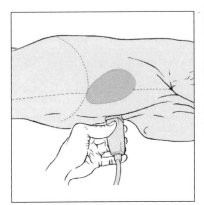

Fig 3.90 Examination in left lateral recumbency

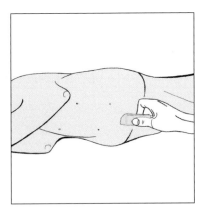

Fig 3.91 Subcostal examination in lateral recumbency

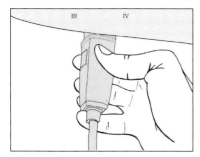

Fig 3.92 Right lateral recumbency parasternal, third–fourth intercostal space position of transducer: upright

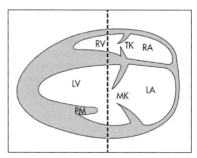

Fig 3.93 Longitudinal axis (four-chamber view) B-Mode

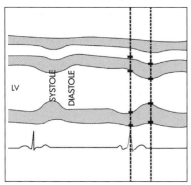

Fig 3.94 Longitudinal axis M-Mode

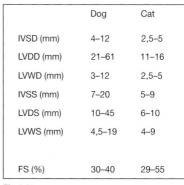

	Dog	Cat
IVSD (mm)	4–12	2,5–5
LVDD (mm)	21–61	11–16
LVWD (mm)	3–12	2,5–5
IVSS (mm)	7–20	5–9
LVDS (mm)	10–45	6–10
LVWS (mm)	4,5–19	4–9
FS (%)	30–40	29–55

Fig 3.95 Measurements longitudinal axis M-/B-Mode

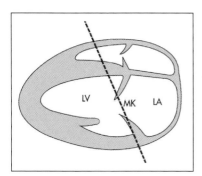

Fig 3.96 Longitudinal axis (mitral valve) B-Mode

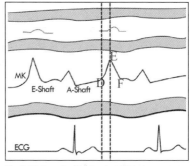

Fig 3.97 Longitudinal axis M-Mode

	Dog	Cat
DEAMP (mm)	17–18	
EPSS (mm)	3–4	2–6
EF-Slope (mm/s)	150–155	55–87

Fig 3.98 Measurements longitudinal axis M-Mode

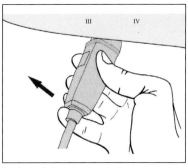

Fig 3.99 Right lateral recumbency parasternal, third–fourth intercostal space, position of transducer: tilt towards cranial

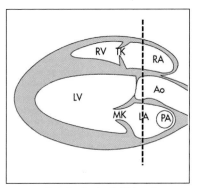

Fig 3.100 Longitudinal axis (LV-outflow tract) B-Mode

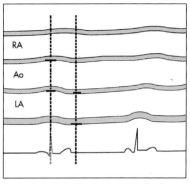

Fig 3.101 Longitudinal axis M-Mode

	Dog	Cat
LA (mm)	12–33	8–15
Ao (mm)	10–30	7–12
LA:Ao	<1,2	<1,2

Fig 3.102 Measurements longitudinal axis M-Mode

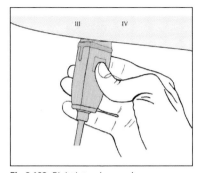

Fig 3.103 Right lateral recumbency parasternal, third–fourth intercostal space, position of Transducer: turn 90° anticlockwise

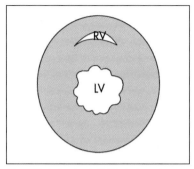

Fig 3.104 Lateral axis B-Mode (apex)

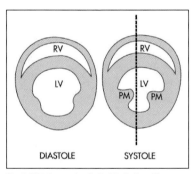

Fig 3.105 Lateral axis B-Mode (papillary muscle plane)

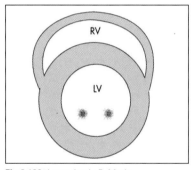

Fig 3.106 Lateral axis B-Mode (chordae plane)

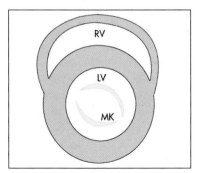

Fig 3.107 Lateral axis B-Mode (mitral valve plane)

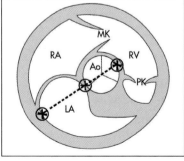

Fig 3.108 Lateral axis B-Mode (pulmonary artery)

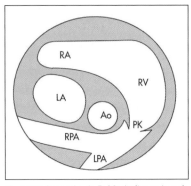

Fig 3.109 Lateral axis B-Mode (heart base)

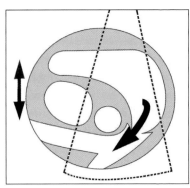

Fig 3.110 Colour-doppler (pulmonary valve)

	Dog	Cat
LA (mm)	12–33	8–15
Ao (mm)	10–30	7–12
LA:Ao	<1,2	<1,2

Fig 3.111 Measurements (LA:Ao)

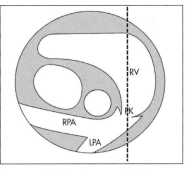

Fig 3.112 CW-doppler measuring line (pulmonary valve) (CW = continuous wave)

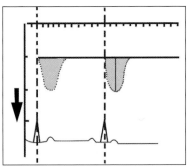

Fig 3.113 CW-doppler (pulmonary valve)

	Dog	Cat
Vmax (m/s)	0,8–1,1	0,9–1,1

Fig 3.114 Measurements CW-doppler (pulmonary valve)

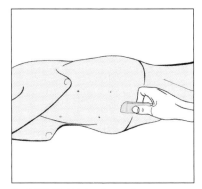

Fig 3.115 Right lateral recumbency: subcostal

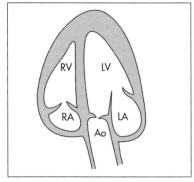

Fig 3.116 Longitudinal axis B-Mode (LV-outflow tract)

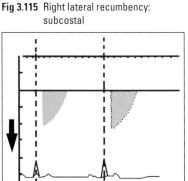

Fig 3.117 Longitudinal axis CW-doppler (aortic valve)

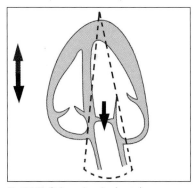

Fig 3.118 Colour-doppler (aorta)

	Dog	Cat
Vmax (m/s)	1,0–1,2	

Fig 3.119 Measurements CW-doppler (aortic valve)

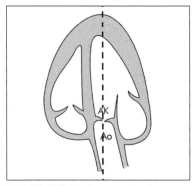

Fig 3.120 CW-doppler measuring line (aortic valve)

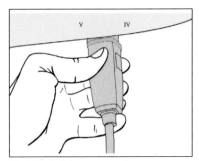

Fig 3.121 Left lateral recumbency: parasternal fourth–fifth intercostal space. Position of transducer: oblique towards the right ear

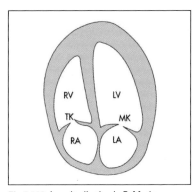

Fig 3.122 Longitudinal axis B-Mode (four-chamber view)

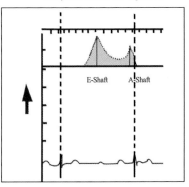

Fig 3.123 CW-doppler (mitral valve)

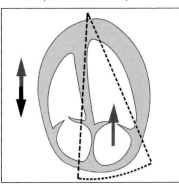

Fig 3.124 Longitudinal axis colour doppler (left heart)

	Dog	Cat
VEL-E (m/s)	0,6–09	
VEL-A (m/s)	0,5–06	
E/A		<1,2
MVA (cm²)	7–8	

Fig 3.125 Measurements CW-doppler (mitral valve)

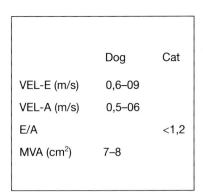

Fig 3.126 CW-doppler measuring line (mitral valve)

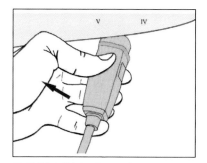

Fig 3.127 Left lateral recumbency: parasternal fourth–fifth intercostal space. Position of transducer: tilt towards cranial

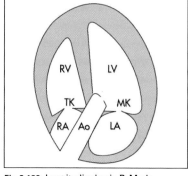

Fig 3.128 Longitudinal axis B-Mode (five-chamber view)

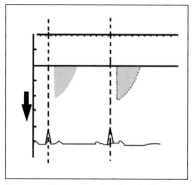

Fig 3.129 CW-doppler (aortic valve)

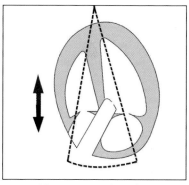

Fig 3.130 Colour-doppler (aorta)

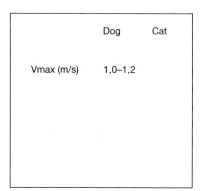

	Dog	Cat
Vmax (m/s)	1,0–1,2	

Fig 3.131 Measurements CW-doppler (aortic valve)

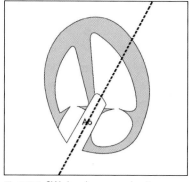

Fig 3.132 CW-doppler measuring line (aortic valve)

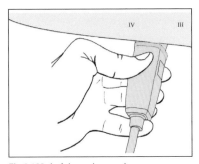

Fig 3.133 Left lateral recumbency: parasternal third–fourth intercostal space. Position of transducer: upright

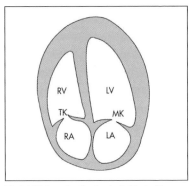

Fig 3.134 Longitudinal axis B-Mode (four-chamber view)

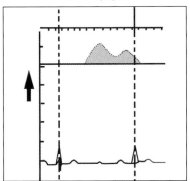

Fig 3.135 CW-doppler (tricuspid valve)

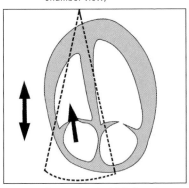

Fig 3.136 Colour-doppler (right heart)

	Dog	Cat
VEL-E (m/s)	0,5–0,8	
VEL-A (m/s)	0,3–0,6	
E/A		<1,1
MVA (cm²)	7–8	

Fig 3.137 Measurements CW-doppler (tricuspid valve)

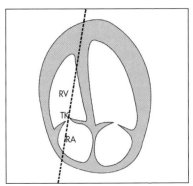

Fig 3.138 CW-doppler measuring line (tricuspid valve)

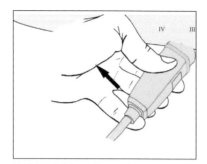

Fig 3.139 Left lateral recumbency: parasternal third–fourth intercostal space. Position of transducer: shallow tilt towards cranial

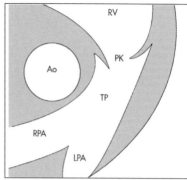

Fig 3.140 Longitudinal axis B-Mode (RV-outflow tract)

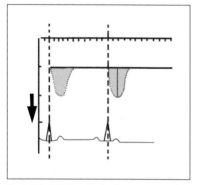

Fig 3.141 CW-doppler (pulmonary artery)

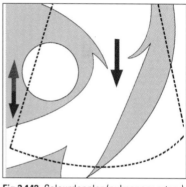

Fig 3.142 Colourdoppler (pulmonary artery)

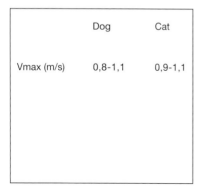

	Dog	Cat
Vmax (m/s)	0,8-1,1	0,9-1,1

Fig 3.143 Measurements CW-doppler (pulmonary valve)

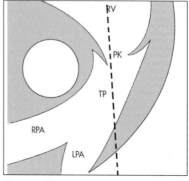

Fig 3.144 CW-doppler measuring line (pulmonary valve)

Method

- **Preparation**
  - Lateral recumbency, ultrasound table with window, net
  - Possibly clipping of fur (ultrasound window left + right thoracic wall + subcostal)
  - Ultrasound contact gel
  - Sector-/doppler transducer 3.5–7.5 MHz

- **Technique**

  Right lateral recumbency
  - Place the transducer parasternal in the third–fourth intercostal space in an upright position
  - Place the transducer parasternal in the third–fourth intercostal space and tilt towards cranial
  - Turn the transducer parasternal in the third–fourth intercostal space anticlockwise by 90° (to right)
  - Position the transducer subcostal

  Left lateral recumbency
  - Place the transducer parasternal in the fourth–fifth intercostal space in an oblique manner facing towards the right ear
  - Place the transducer parasternal in the fourth–fifth intercostal space and tilt towards cranial
  - Hold the transducer upright parasternal in the third–fourth intercostal space
  - Hold the transducer parasternal in the third–fourth intercostal space and tilt towards cranial

Echocardiography Findings

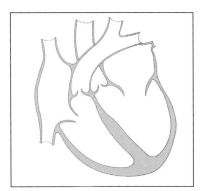

Fig 3.145 Dilated cardiomyopathy (Vmax mitral valve/ aorta)

Dilated cardiomyopathy

2D   – LV ± RV thinning of the myocardium
    – hypokinesia (LV + septum)
    – paradoxical septum movement
    – LA ± RA dilatation
    – possibly thrombi, pericardial effusion

M-Mode – FS ↓
    – LA: Ao
    – EPSS, E/A

Colour doppler
    – Mitral valve insufficiency (regurgitation)

CW-doppler

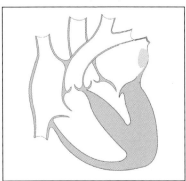

3.146 Hypertrophic cardiomyopathy

Hypertrophic cardiomyopathy

2D   – LV thickening of the myocardium
    – septal thickening
    – hyperkinesia (LV + septum)
    – LA dilation
    – possibly thrombi, pericardial effusion

M-Mode – FS
    – LA:Ao
    – DEAMP , EPSS ↓, E/A ↓

Colour-doppler
    – possibly mitral valve regurgitation

CW-Doppler
    – Vmax mitral valve ↓

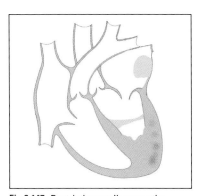

Fig 3.147 Restrictive cardiomyopathy

Restrictive cardiomyopathy

2D   – apical LV thickening of myocardium
    – LA + RA dilation
    – Septal thickening
    – endo-/myocardial fibrosis (moderator bands)
    – possibly RV hypertrophy/dilation

M-Mode – LA: Ao
    – Colour-doppler
    – mitral valve insufficiency (regurgitation)

CW-Doppler
    – Vmax mitral valve ↓

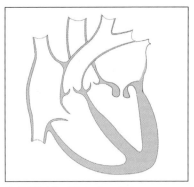

Fig 3.148 Mitral Valve Insufficiency

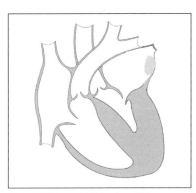

Fig 3.149 Tricuspid Valve Insufficiency

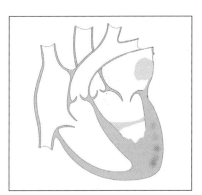

Fig 3.150 Subaortic Stenosis

Mitral Valve Insufficiency

2D	– Thickening of mitral valve or prolapse/ tendinous cord rupture
	– LA dilation
	– possibly LV hypertrophy/dilation
	– hyperkinesia (septum)
M-Mode	– LA:Ao
	– DEAMP, EF-slope
Colour-Doppler	
	– Mitral valve regurgitation (turbulences)
CW-Doppler	
	– Vmax mitral valve (up to 5–6m/s)

Tricuspid Valve Insufficiency

2D	– thickening of the tricuspid valve
	– RA dilation
	– RV dilation
	– Paradoxical septal movement
M-Mode	– LA:Ao
	– DEAMP , EF-slope
Colour-Doppler	
	– tricuspid valve regurgitation (turbulences)
CW-Doppler	
	– Vmax tricuspid valve (< 2 m/s)

Subaortic Stenosis

2D	– subvalvular fibrous ring
	– poststenotic aortic dilation
	– LV myocardial thickening
	– possibly myocardial scars
M-Mode	
Colour-Doppler	
	– aortic turbulences
	– possibly mitral valve insufficiency
CW-Doppler	
	– Vmax aortic valve

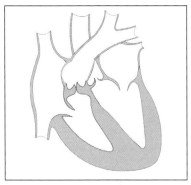

Fig 3.151 Pulmonary stenosis

Pulmonary stenosis

2D   – thickening of the pulmonary valve
 – RV myocardial thickening
 – poststenotic dilation of pulmonary artery
 – paradoxical septal movement

M-Mode

Colour doppler
 – turbulences pulmonary artery
 – possibly tricuspid valve insufficiency (regurgitation)

CW-doppler
 – Vmax pulmonary valve (> 2 m/s)

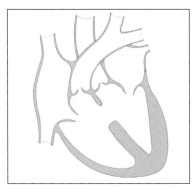

Fig 3.152 Ventricular septal defect

Ventricular septal defect

2D   – septal defect

M-Mode

Colour doppler
 – turbulences
 – possibly regurgitation of aortic valve
 – shunt direction (L–R, R–L)

CW-Doppler
 – shunt direction (L–R, R–L)

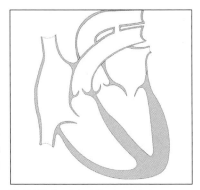

Fig 3.153 Persistent Ductus Arteriosus

Persistent Ductus Arteriosus

2D   – aortic dilation
 – dilation of pulmonary artery
 – ductus
 – myocardial thinning of LA + LV
 – paradoxical septal movement

M-Mode – FS Ø

Colour doppler
 – shunt direction (L–R, R–L)
 – possibly pulmonary insufficiency
 – possibly mitral valve insufficiency

CW-doppler
 – Vmax aorta

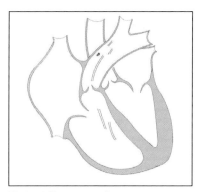

Fig 3.154 Heart worm disease (dirofilariosis)

Heart worm disease

2D   – dilation of pulmonary artery
      – myocardial thinning of RA + RV
      – poststenotic dilation of pulmonary artery
      – paradoxical septal movement
      – heart worms (TP, RV, RA)
      – possibly thrombi
M-Mode
Colour-Doppler
      – possibly tricuspid valve insufficiency (regurgitation)
      – possibly stenosis/insufficiency of pulmonary artery

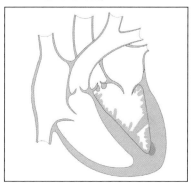

Fig 3.155 Endo-/myocarditis

Endo-/myocarditis

2D   – endo-/ myocardial fibrinous coating
Colour doppler
      – Possibly mitral valve insufficiency
      – Possibly aortic valve insufficiency

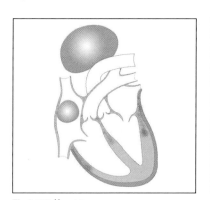

Fig 3.156 Heart tumours

Heart tumours

2D   – heart base tumour (chemodectoma)
      – haemangiosarcoma
      – pericardial mass (mesothelioma)
      – lymphosarcoma (cat)

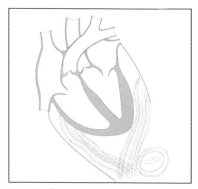

Fig 3.157 Peritoneopericardial diaphragmatic hernia

Peritoneopericardial diaphragmatic hernia

2D   –   pericardium contains small intestines ± spleen

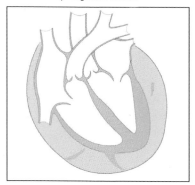

Fig 3.158 Pericardial effusion

Pericardial effusion

2D   –   fluid filled space between peri- and epicardium
        –   possibly thickening of the pericardium
        –   possibly fibrin/thrombi
        –   swinging heart movement

Findings

- **Physiological**
  - Nothing abnormal to detect (NAD)

- **Pathological**

  ### Acquired heart diseases
  - Dilated cardiomyopathy (DCMP)
  - Hypertrophic cardiomyopathy (HCMP)
  - Restrictive cardiomyopathy (RCMP)
  - Mitral valve insufficiency (MI)
  - Tricuspid valve insufficiency (TI)
  - Endo-/myocarditis
  - Right-sided cardiac enlargement (cor pulmonale)
  - Heart worm disease (dirofilariosis)
  - Heart tumours
  - Pericardial effusion
  - Atrial thrombi
  - Atrial rupture
  - Rupture of the tendinous cords
  - Peritoneopericardial diaphragmatic hernia

  ### Congenital heart diseases
  - (Sub-)aortic stenosis (SAS)
  - Pulmonary stenosis (PS)
  - Persistent ductus arteriosus (PDA)
  - Ventricular septal defect (VSD)
  - Atrial septal defect (ASD)
  - Tetralogy of Fallot

Blood Pressure Measurement

Indication

- Suspected hypertension (kidney, heart or CNS-disease, hyphaema, mydriasis, diabetes mellitus, hyperthyroidism, Cushing's disease)

Oscillometric Blood Pressure Measuring

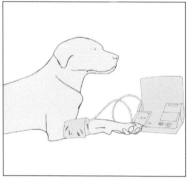

Fig 3.159 Blood Pressure Measuring

Normal values – dog

Systolic:	144±27 (mmHg)
Diastolic:	91±20 (mmHg)
Average:	110±21 (mmHg)

Normal values – cat

Systolic:	117–149 (mmHg)
Diastolic:	48–102 (mmHg)
Average:	61–124 (mmHg)

Method

- **Technique**
  - Apply the cuff
    - dog (radial artery – lower leg)
    - cat (brachial artery – upper leg)
  - Turn on the machine
  - Press start
  - Repeat (2–3 times)

Findings

- **Physiological**
  - Nothing abnormal to detect (NAD)

- **Pathological**
  - Hypertension (kidney failure, heart failure, hyperthyroidism, diabetes mellitus, Cushing's disease, CNS disease)

Measuring the Central Venous Pressure

Indication

- Monitoring as part of intravenous fluid therapy
- Cardiological intensive care monitoring

Measuring the Central Venous Pressure (CVP)

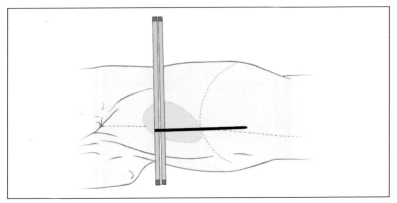

Fig 3.160 Determine the zero point (sternum)

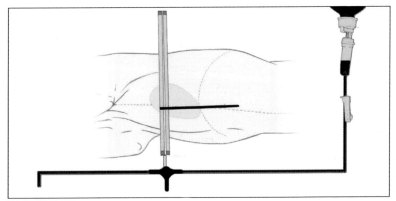

Fig 3.161 Vent the system

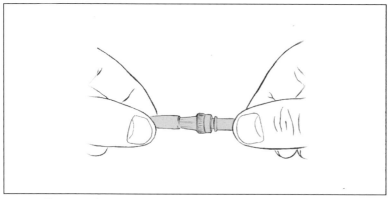

Fig 3.162 Connect to the central venous catheter

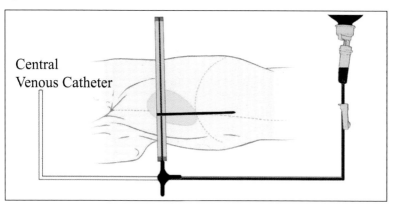

Central
Venous Catheter

Fig 3.163 Fill up the pressure gauge

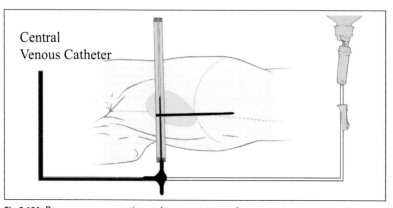

Central
Venous Catheter

Fig 3.164 Pressure compensation and pressure measuring

Method

- **Preparation**
  - Central venous catheter
  - Sternal position or lateral recumbency
  - System: Medifix®, Braun

- **Technique**

  Pressure gauge positioning
  - Attach the pressure gauge outside on the cage door

  Determine zero point
  - Pointer orientation
  - Sternal position: third intercostal space at the chondrocostal junction
  - Lateral recumbency: sternum

  Fill up the system
  - Open the three-way tap
    Infusion bag to central venous catheter
  - Vent
  - Connect the infusion line to the central venous catheter
  - Open the three-way tap
    Infusion bag to pressure gauge
  - Fill up the pressure gauge
  - Open the three-way tap
    Pressure gauge to central venous catheter
  - Measure the water column

Findings

- **Physiological**
  - 1 bis +5 mm H_2O

- **Pathological**
  - Hypertension (volume overload)
  - Hypotension (volume deficit)

Thoracocentesis

Indication

- Pleural effusion of unknown origin

Thoracocentesis

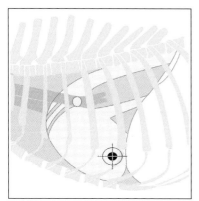

Fig 3.165 Puncture site

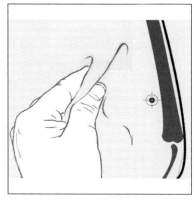

Fig 3.166 Puncture of the thorax cranial of the rib

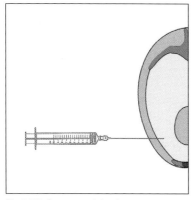

Fig 3.167 Puncture of the thorax

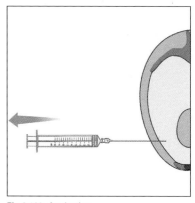

Fig 3.168 Aspiration

Method

- **Preparation**
  - While standing on the examination table clip fur and disinfect skin (left/right thoracic wall)
  - System: 10ml syringe with three-way-tap and attached cannula

- **Technique**
  - Puncture site: cranial of the rib in seventh–eighth intercostal space, dorsal (if pneumothorax), ventral (if pleural effusion)
  - Push the skin to cranial
  - Puncture the thoracic wall slowly
  - Aspirate air/fluid until negative pressure has been created
  - Possibly close the three-way tap, change the syringe, open three-way tap again and repeat aspiration
  - Remove the puncture needle while maintaining insertion angle
  - Let go of the skin that was previously moved forward
  - Compress the puncture site (2–5 min)
  - Examine/process the sample
  - Take control radiographs

Complications

- Thoracic haemorrhage (rib vessels, lung puncture)
- Pneumothorax (lung puncture, leak)
- Subcutaneous emphysema
- Infection

Pericardiocentesis

Indication

- Pericardial effusion

Pericardiocentesis

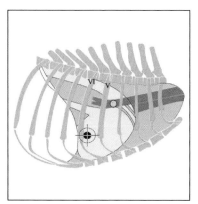

Fig 3.169 Puncture site

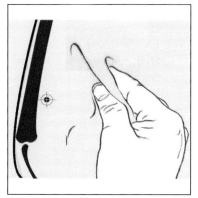

Fig 3.170 Puncture of the thorax cranial of the rib

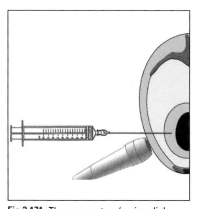

Fig 3.171 Thorax puncture/pericardial puncture

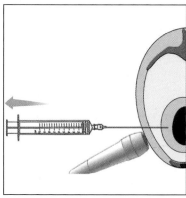

Fig 3.172 Aspiration

Method

- **Preparation**
  - Position: left lateral recumbency, sternal, possibly standing
  - Clip fur and disinfect skin
  - System: venous catheter, three-way tap, syringe
  - ECG-control
  - Ultrasound-control

- **Technique**
  - Push the skin over the puncture site towards cranial
  - Pericardial puncture
  - Right thoracic wall, fifth intercostal space, cranial of the rib near the chondrocostal junction
  - Horizontal puncture while lightly aspirating
  - Drainage: change the syringe after closure of the three-way-tap
  - Remove the puncture cannula and compress the puncture site
  - Check if the aspirate is coagulating: no coagulation in case of a pericardial effusion (coagulation in case of cardiac puncture)
  - Take control radiographs

Complications

- Haemorrhage
- Pneumothorax
- Ventricular ectopic complexes
- Heart perforation
- Lung perforation
- Infection
- Recurrence

Abdominocentesis

Indication

* Abdominal effusion

Abdominocentesis

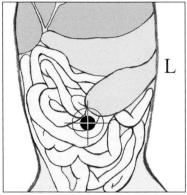

Fig 3.173 Puncture site

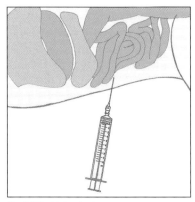

Fig 3.174 Abdominal puncture

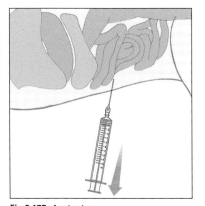

Fig 3.175 Aspiration

Method

- **Preparation**
  - Lateral recumbency
  - Clip fur and disinfect skin

- **Technique**
  - Possible evacuation of urinary bladder required
  - Puncture the abdominal wall paramedian and caudal of the umbilicus (syringe with attached hypodermic needle)
  - Direction of puncture towards caudal
  - Aspirate
  - Remove the syringe and needle

Complications

- Splenic puncture
- Intestinal puncture
- Puncture of urinary bladder
- Peritonitis

Further Cardiological Examination Methods

- Laboratory investigations
- Angiography

4 Respiratory Examination Methods

Case History

Principal Symptoms

- Nasal discharge
- Sneezing
- Coughing
- Respiratory distress
- Stridor
- Stertor
- Cyanosis

Inspection

Indication

- Part of the general examination

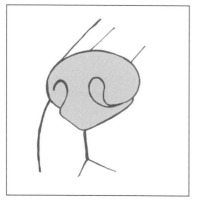

Fig 4.1 Inspection of the nostrils

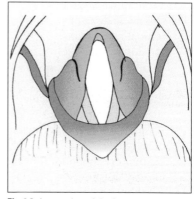

Fig 4.2 Inspection of the larynx

Method

- **Technique**
  - Observe the body posture/stance and respiration at rest
  - Observe the nostrils, larynx, neck, thorax and abdomen on the examination table (often combined with palpation)
- **Evaluation criteria**
  - Size, shape, symmetry, colour, rhythm

Findings

- **Physiological**
  - Costoabdominal respiration/respiration rate 10–30/min
- **Pathological**

  Respiration
  - Abdominal respiration (thoracic disease)
  - Costal respiration (abdominal disease)
  - Bradypnoea (sedation, CNS disease)
  - Tachypnoea (excitement, pain, systemic disease)
  - Inspiratory dyspnoea (upper airway disease)
  - Expiratory dyspnoea (lower airway disease)
  - Orthopnoea (lower airway disease)
  - Open mouth breathing (lower airway disease)
  - Cheyne-Stokes breathing (CNS disease, heart or endocrine disease)

Body posture/stance
  - Dyspnoea: broad-legged, standing or in sternal position, mydriasis

Nostrils
  - Narrowing of the nostril (brachycephalic syndrome)
  - Nasal discharge (uni- or bilateral)
  - Hyperkeratinisation/ depigmentation of the nasal plane
  - Inflamed mucocutaneous junctions
  - Tumour
  - Foreign body
  - Lesions caused by trauma

Larynx/pharynx
  - Laryngitis
  - Laryngospasm
  - Laryngeal paralysis (uni-/bilateral)
  - Glottal oedema
  - Nasopharyngeal tumour
  - Nasopharyngeal foreign body
  - Tonsillitis/peritonsillar abscess/tonsillar tumour
  - Oronasal fistula/cleft palate
  - Lesions caused by trauma

Throat/Thorax
  - Injuries caused by trauma
  - Subcutaneous emphysema

Abdomen
  - Injuries caused by trauma
  - Increased abdominal girth

Palpation

Indication

- Part of the general examination

Palpation

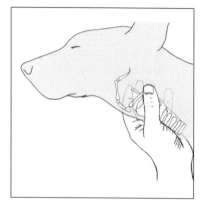

Fig 4.3 Palpation of the larynx and trachea

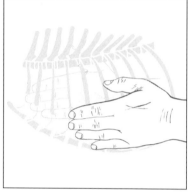

Fig 4.4 Palpation of the thorax

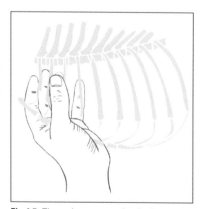

Fig 4.5 Thoracic compression in the cat

Method

- **Technique**
  - Touch the larynx, trachea, thoracic wall and abdomen
- **Evaluation criteria**
  - Size, shape, symmetry, consistency, temperature, painfulness, cough

Findings

- **Physiological**
  - Nothing abnormal to detect (NAD)
- **Pathological**

  Larynx
  - Urge to cough (laryngitis)
  - Tumour
  - Foreign body
  - Injury caused by trauma

Trachea / throat
- Urge to cough (tracheitis/tracheo-bronchitis)
- Subcutaneous emphysema/rupture of the trachea
- Goitre
- Tumour
- Injury caused by trauma

Thorax
- Reduced compression/elasticity of the cranial thorax in the cat (mediastinal disease)
- Tumour
- Injury caused by trauma (intercostal muscles/ribs)

Percussion

Indication

- Respiratory disease

Percussion

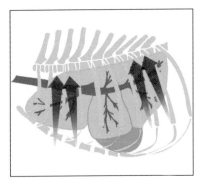

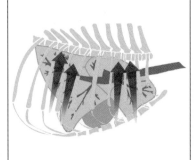

Fig 4.6 Percussion areas of the left thoracic wall

Fig 4.7 Percussion areas of the right thoracic wall

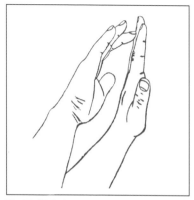

Fig 4.8 Digital percussion technique

Method

- **Technique**
  - Tap against each side of the thoracic wall
  - Indirect percussion: middle finger taps onto the middle phalanx of the other middle finger

- **Evaluation criteria**
  - Sound qualities of each side in comparison

Findings

- **Physiological**
  - Sonorous
  - Sound quality: loud, low, long

- **Pathological**

  Hypersonorous / subtympanic
  - Sound quality: louder, lower, longer (pulmonary emphysema, pneumothorax)

  Dullness / muffles
  - Sound quality: quiet, high, short (pleural effusion, pneumonia, atelectasis, tumour)

Auscultation

Indication

- Part of the general examination

Auscultation

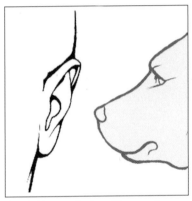

Fig 4.9 Listen to the breathing sounds

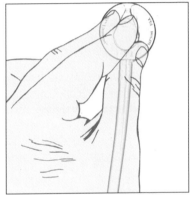

Fig 4.10 Auscultation with a stethoscope

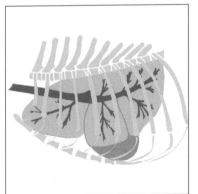

Fig 4.11 Auscultation areas of the left thoracic wall

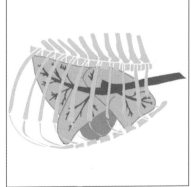

Fig 4.12 Auscultation areas of the right thoracic wall

Method

- **Technique**
  - Listen to the lung sounds in the standing patient and compare both sides with each other
  - Listen to the tracheal sounds over its whole length
- **Evaluation criteria**
  - Sound qualities

Findings

- **Physiological**

  Bronchovesicular breathing sound
  - Mixed sound consisting of:
    1. Vesicular breathing: quiet, low frequency, loud during inspiration
    2. Bronchial breathing: loud, high frequency, louder during expiration

- **Pathological**

  Stridor
  - Loud inspiratory stenotic sound (upper airways stenosis)

  Stertor
  - Snoring (overlong soft palate/tonsillar disease/tumour)

  Wet breathing sounds
  - Rattling noises (fine/coarse) louder during inspiration (pulmonary oedema, bronchopneumonia)

  Dry breathing sounds
  - Wheezing, humming, whistling (obstructive bronchitis)

  Quiet/missing breathing sounds
  - Pulmonary atelectasis, pulmonary emphysema, thoracic effusion, tumour

  Pleural rubbing sounds
  - Dry rubbing sounds in time with the breathing (pleuritis)

Complications

- Panting/purring

X-Ray Study

Indication

- Respiratory disease

X-Ray Study

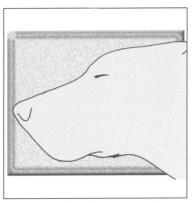

Fig 4.13 Lateral positioning to view the nasal passage

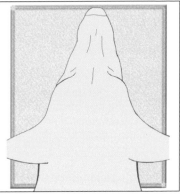

Fig 4.14 Positioning to view the nasal passage (dorsoventral view)

Fig 4.15 Positioning with intraoral plate

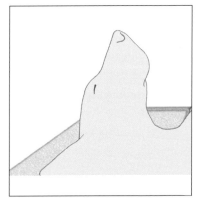

Fig 4.16 Positioning to view the sinuses

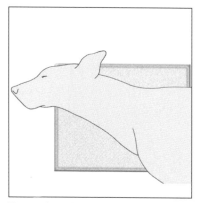

Fig 4.17 Lateral positioning to view the larynx and throat

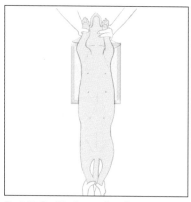

Fig 4.18 Positioning to view the trachea/thorax (ventrodorsal view)

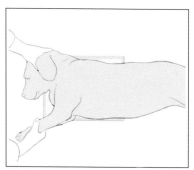

Fig 4.19 Right lateral positioning for the thoracic view

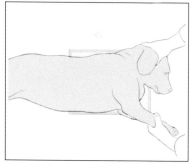

Fig 4.20 Left lateral positioning for the thoracic view

Method

- **Technique**
  - Perform risk/benefit assessment (if the patient is dyspnoeic)
  - Plan and agree the proposed procedure with colleagues and owners
  - Fully inform the owner (consider questions about pregnancy and age range)
  - Handle the patient calmly and in a coordinated manner
  - Possible distraction
  - Projection of two views if at all possible

Radiological Findings

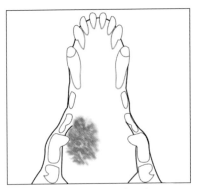

Fig 4.21 Tumour of the nasal cavity

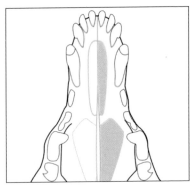

Fig 4.22 Sinusitis

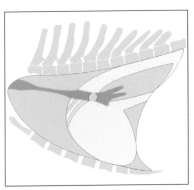

Fig 4.23 Tracheal collapse

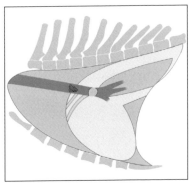

Fig 4.24 Tracheal foreign body

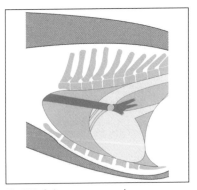

Fig 4.25 Subcutaneous emphysema

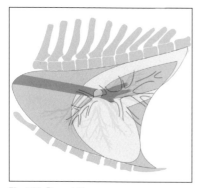

Fig 4.26 Bronchitis

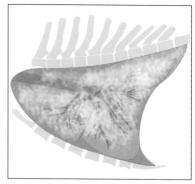

Fig 4.27 Pneumonia

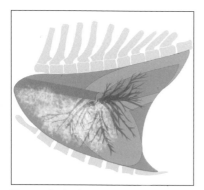

Fig 4.28 Aspiration pneumonia

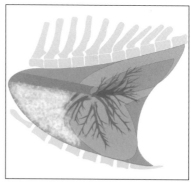

Fig 4.29 Pulmonary contusion

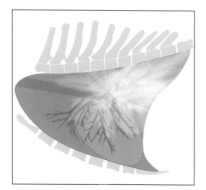

Fig 4.30 Pulmonary oedema

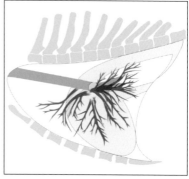

Fig 4.31 Pulmonary emphysema

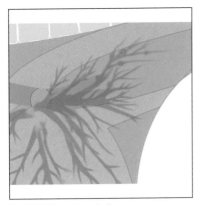

Fig 4.32 Thromboembolism

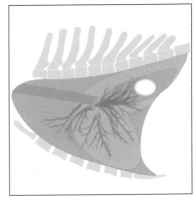

Fig 4.33 Pulmonary tumour

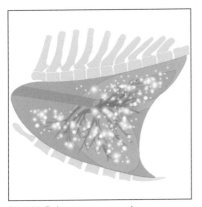

Fig 4.34 Pulmonary metastasis

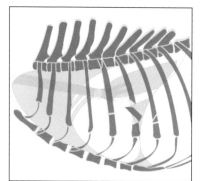

Fig 4.35 Rib fracture

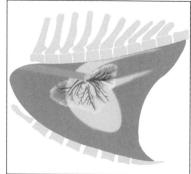

Fig 4.36 Pneumothorax

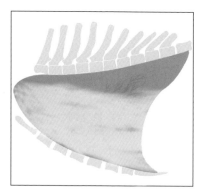

Fig 4.37 Thoracic effusion

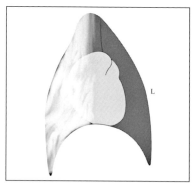

Fig 4.38 Unilateral thoracic effusion

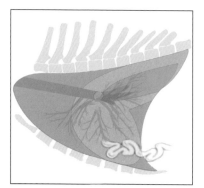

Fig 4.39 Diaphragmatic hernia

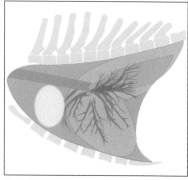

Fig 4.40 Thymoma

Findings

- **Physiological**
  - Nothing abnormal to detect (NAD)

- **Pathological**

  Nasal passage and sinuses
  - Foreign bodies
  - Tumour of the nasal cavity
  - Radiopacity (inflammation/secretion) (sinusitis/rhinitis)
  - Dental abscess/oronasal fistula

  Trachea
  - Tracheal collapse
  - Tracheal hypoplasia
  - Tracheal stenosis
  - Foreign body
  - Tumour
  - Subcutaneous emphysema/tracheal rupture
  - Elevation of the trachea (cardiomegaly/mediastinal mass)

  Lung
  - Bronchitis/feline asthma
  - Bronchopneumonia
  - Pneumonia (alveolar/interstitial pattern)
  - Aspiration pneumonia
  - Pulmonary haemorrhage/contusion
  - Pulmonary oedema (cardiogenic/non-cardiogenic)
  - Pulmonary atelectasis
  - Pulmonary emphysema/bullous emphysema
  - Thromboembolism
  - Dilation of pulmonary vessels
  - Right-sided cardiomegaly/cor pulmonale
  - Pulmonary abscess
  - Tumour
  - Foreign body
  - Lung lobe torsion
  - Calcification
  - Pulmonary metastasis

  Thorax
  - Rib fracture
  - Pneumothorax
  - Pneumomediastinum
  - Thoracic effusion/unilateral thoracic effusion
  - Mediastinal mass
  - Heart base tumour
  - Lymphadenopathy
  - Diaphragmatic hernia
  - Thymoma

Complications

- Traumatic injuries on the X-ray table
- Respiratory arrest (in case of dyspnoea)
- Radiation exposure

Endoscopy

Indication

- Upper airway disease of unknown origin, tissue sample (biopsy)

Rhinoscopy

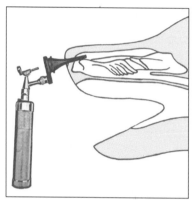

Fig 4.41 Rhinoscopy via an otoscope

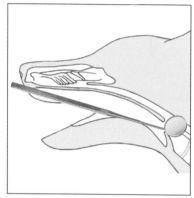

Fig 4.42 Retrograde rhinoscopy via a dental mirror

Rhinoscopy: Rigid Endoscope

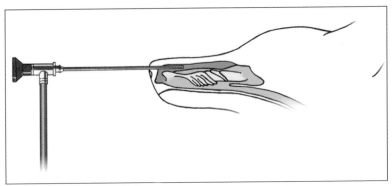

Fig 4.43 Rhinoscopy with a rigid endoscope (dorsal nasal passage)

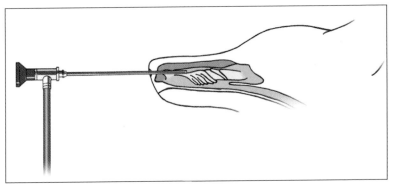

Fig 4.44 Rhinoscopy with a rigid endoscope (middle nasal passage)

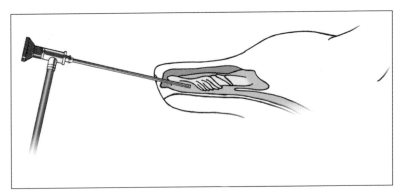

Fig 4.45 Rhinoscopy with a rigid endoscope (ventral nasal passage)

Rhinoscopy: Flexible Endoscope

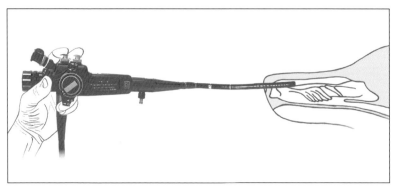

Fig 4.46 Rhinoscopy with a flexible endoscope (orthograde rhinoscopy)

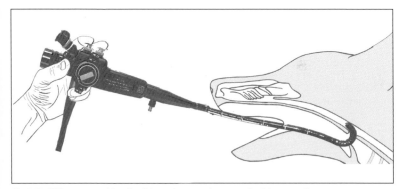

Fig 4.47 Rhinoscopy with a flexible endoscope (retrograde rhinoscopy)

Method

- **Preparation**
    - Sedation/general anaesthesia
    - Sternal position, support the head with a sand bag
    - Endotracheal intubation
    - Insert some cotton wool soaked in nephazoline nitrate intranasally (2–3 min) to assist the reduction of mucous membrane swelling

- **Technique**

    Orthograde rhinoscopy
    - Rhinoscopy of the dorsal/middle/ventral nasal passage (entrance through the nostril)

    Retrograde rhinoscopy
    - Rhinoscopy of the nasopharynx (entrance orally)
    - Insert the flexible endoscope through the mouth
    - Retroflex the endoscope
    - Pull the endoscope back and by doing so insert into the nasopharynx underneath the soft palate

- **Evaluation criteria**
    - Size, shape, symmetry, colour

Findings

- **Physiological**
    - Nothing abnormal to detect (NAD)

- **Pathological**
    - Nasal discharge (uni- or bilateral) (haemorrhage/epistaxis, purulent, muculent, serous)
    - foreign body (e.g., awns/grass seeds in the dog, grass blades in the cat)
    - rhinitis (purulent, serous, aspergillosis in the dog)
    - tumour
    - nasopharyngeal polyp (cat)

Complications

- Haemorrhage
- Swelling of mucous membranes

Laryngoscopy

Indication

- Upper airway disease of unknown origin
- Stridor, stertor, retching, voice alteration, endotracheal intubation

Laryngoscopy

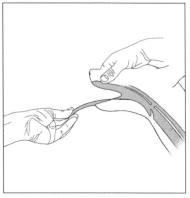

Fig 4.48 Holding technique to perform laryngoscopy

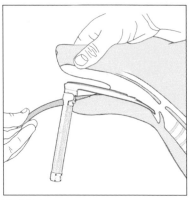

Fig 4.49 Laryngoscopy

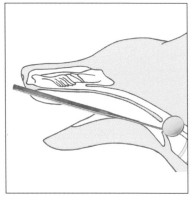

Fig 4.50 Laryngoscopy with a dental mirror

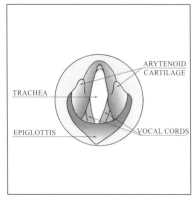

Fig 4.51 Larynx

ARYTENOID CARTILAGE

TRACHEA

EPIGLOTTIS

VOCAL CORDS

Method

- **Preparation**
    - Sedation/general anaesthesia
    - Sternal position with an elevated head and pulled out tongue (possibly lateral position)
    - Laryngoscope, endoscope, spatula + light source or dental mirror + light source

- **Technique**
    - Open the mouth
    - Pull out the tongue
    - Press down the base of the tongue with the spatula of the laryngoscope
    - Observe the pharynx and larynx without touching the glottis
    - Consider pulling back the soft palate with a spey hook if required

- **Evaluation criteria**
    - Size, shape, symmetry, position, function (inspiration/expiration), colour

Findings

- **Physiological**
    - Nothing abnormal to detect (NAD)

- **Pathological**
    - Glottal oedema
    - Laryngitis
    - Foreign body
    - Tumour
    - Laryngeal collapse
    - Laryngeal spasm
    - Hyperplasia of the vestibular folds
    - Laryngeal paralysis (recurrent laryngeal nerve paresis) (uni- or bilateral)

Complications

- Laryngospasm

Tracheo-/Bronchoscopy

Indication

- Lower airway disease of unknown origin, tissue sample (biopsy)
- Tracheobronchitis of unknown origin

Bronchoscopy: flexible endoscope

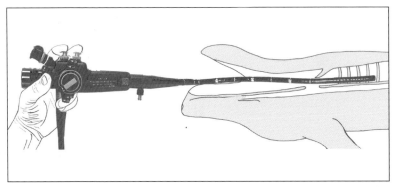

Fig 4.52 Insert the flexible endoscope through the mouth

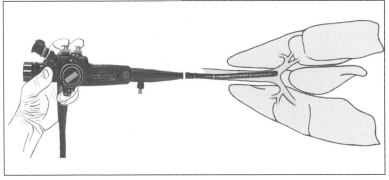

Fig 4.53 Illustration of the trachea and bronchi

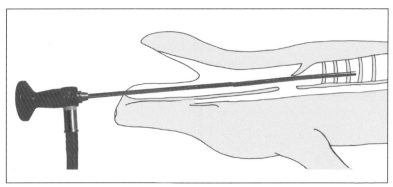

Fig 4.54 Tracheo-/bronchoscopy with a rigid endoscope

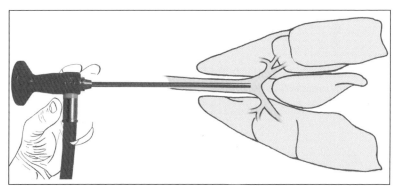

Fig 4.55 Illustration of the bronchi

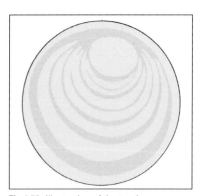

Fig 4.56 Illustration of the trachea

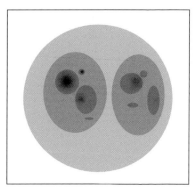

Fig 4.57 Illustration of the bronchi (bifurcation)

Method

- **Preparation**
  - Sedation/general anaesthesia
  - Dorsal position with an extended neck
  - Mouth gag
  - Topical anaesthesia of the glottis (lidocaine 2 per cent spray)

- **Technique**
  - Insert the endoscope carefully under visual control over the epiglottis and into the trachea
  - Suction of secretion as required

- **Evaluation criteria**
  - Size, shape, symmetry, mucous membrane colour

Findings

- **Physiological**
  - Nothing abnormal to detect (NAD)

- **Pathological**
  - Tracheitis/tracheobronchitis
  - Tracheal collapse
  - Tracheal hypoplasia
  - Tracheal stenosis/stricture
  - Foreign body
  - Tumour
  - Pulmonary oedema
  - Pulmonary haemorrhage
  - Tracheal rupture
  - Lung lobe torsion
  - Parasites (lung worm-*Filaroides osleri*)

Complications

- Haemorrhage
- Tracheal/bronchial perforation

Biopsy of the Nasal Mucosa

Indication

- Rhinitis of unknown origin

Biopsy of the Nasal Mucosa

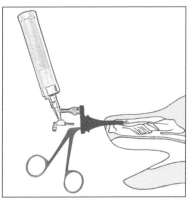

Fig 4.58 Biopsy with an otoscope + biopsy forceps

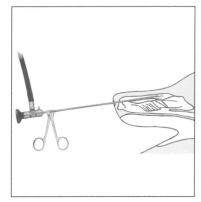

Fig 4.59 Biopsy with a rigid biopsy endoscope

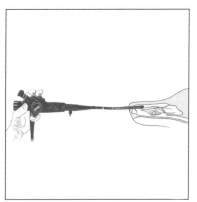

Fig 4.60 Biopsy with a flexible endoscope

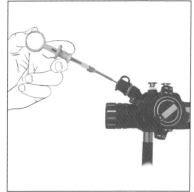

Fig 4.61 Insert the biopsy forceps into the biopsy channel of the endoscope

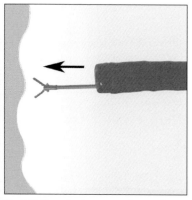

Fig 4.62 Open the forceps and grasp the mucosa

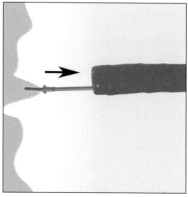

Fig 4.63 Close the forceps and pull them back with a sudden jerk

Method

- **Preparation**
  - In continuation of rhinoscopy

- **Technique**
  - Localisation the biopsy area with the endoscope
  - Insert the biopsy forceps into the biopsy channel of the endoscope
  - Open the biopsy forceps
  - Grasp a piece of mucosa
  - Close the forceps
  - Pull the forceps back with a sudden jerk
  - Remove the forceps through the biopsy channel of the endoscope
  - Transfer the sample via a sterile hypodermic needle into a fixative solution
  - Check the biopsied area with the endoscope

Complications

- Haemorrhage

Biopsy of the Tracheal/Bronchial Mucosa

Indication

- Tracheobronchitis of unknown origin

Biopsy of the Tracheal/Bronchial Mucosa

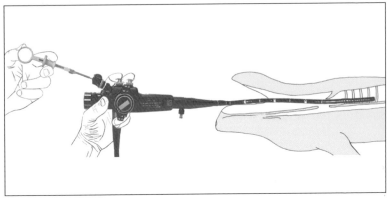

Fig 4.64 Insert the forceps into the biopsy channel of the flexible endoscope

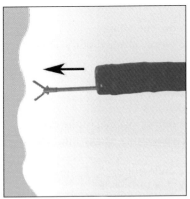

Fig 4.65 Open the forceps and grasp the mucosa

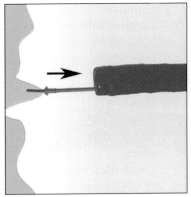

Fig 4.66 Close the forceps and pull them back with a sudden jerk

Method

- **Preparation**
  - In continuation of tracheo-/bronchoscopy

- **Technique**
  - Localise the biopsy area with the endoscope
  - Insert the biopsy forceps into the biopsy channel of the endoscope
  - Open the forceps
  - Grasp the mucosa
  - Close the forceps
  - Pull the forceps back with a sudden jerk
  - Remove the forceps through the biopsy channel of the endoscope
  - Transfer the sample via a sterile hypodermic needle into a fixative solution
  - Check the biopsied area with the endoscope

Complications

- Haemorrhage

Biopsy of the Lung

Indication

- Pneumonia of unknown origin

Transbronchial Biopsy of the Lung

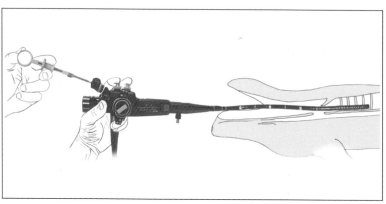

Fig 4.67 Insert the biopsy forceps into biopsy channel of the flexible endoscope

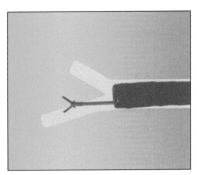

Fig 4.68 Transbronchial biopsy of the lung with the biopsy forceps

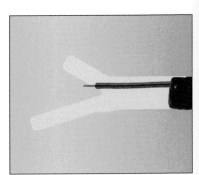

Fig 4.69 Transbronchial fine needle aspiration biopsy

Method

- **Preparation**
  - In continuation of tracheo-/bronchoscopy

- **Technique**

  Transbronchial biopsy of the lung (biopsy forceps)
  - Insert the endoscope as far as possible into the bronchiole
  - Insert the biopsy forceps as far as possible into the biopsy channel of the endoscope
  - Open the forceps
  - Grasp the mucosa
  - Close the forceps
  - Pull the forceps back with a sudden jerk
  - Remove the forceps through the biopsy channel of the endoscope
  - Transfer the sample via a sterile hypodermic needle into a fixative solution
  - Check the biopsied area with the endoscope
  - Take control radiographs

  Transbronchial biopsy of the lung (fine needle aspiration biopsy)
  - Insert the endoscope as far as possible into the bronchiole
  - Insert the biopsy needle as far as possible into the biopsy channel of the endoscope
  - Aspirate
  - Remove the needle through the biopsy channel
  - Transfer the sample onto a microscope slide
  - Check the biopsied area with the endoscope
  - Take control radiographs

Complications

- Haemorrhage
- Pneumothorax
- Pulmonary emphysema
- Pneumonia

Transthoracic Biopsy of the Lung

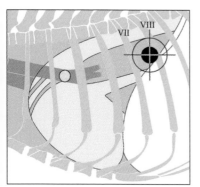

Fig 4.70 Puncture site

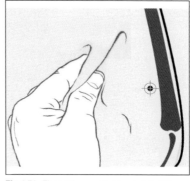

Fig 4.71 Thoracic puncture cranial of the rib

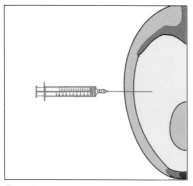

Fig 4.72 Thoracic puncture/ puncture of the lung

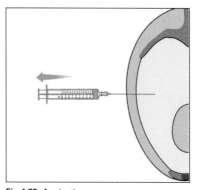

Fig 4.73 Aspiration

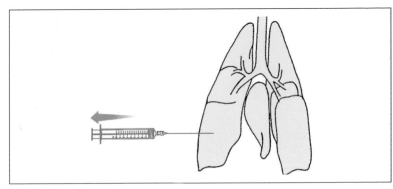

Fig 4.74 Puncture of the caudal lung lobe

Method

- **Preparation**
  - Sedation
  - Clip fur, disinfect skin

- **Technique**
  - Puncture site cranial of eighth rib in seventh–eighth intercostal space, dorsal or according to X-ray finding (two views)
  - Required equipment: 10ml syringe with an attached three-way tap and spinal cannula
  - Push the skin towards cranial
  - Puncture the thoracic wall slowly
  - Readjust the puncture direction
  - Rapidly puncture and immediately aspirate the lung
  - Remove the puncture needle while maintaining the insertion angle
  - Let go of the skin that was previously pushed forwards
  - Compress the puncture site (c. 5 min)
  - Process the sample
  - Take control radiographs

Complications

- Haemorrhage
- Pneumothorax
- Pulmonary emphysema
- Pneumonia

Endotracheal Lavage

Indication

- Tracheobronchitis of unknown origin
- Pneumonia of unknown origin

Tracheo-Bronchial Lavage (TBL)/Broncho-Alveolar Lavage (BAL)

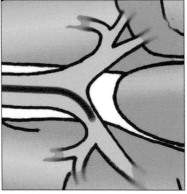

Fig 4.75 Tracheo-bronchial lavage (TBL)

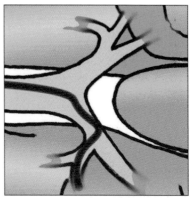

Fig 4.76 Broncho-alveolar lavage (BAL)

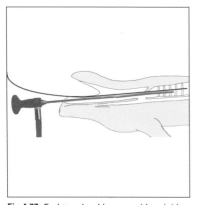

Fig 4.77 Endotracheal lavage with a rigid endoscope

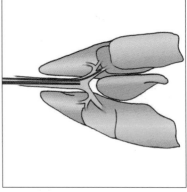

Fig 4.78 Endotracheal lavage with a rigid endoscope

Method

- **Preparation**
  - Sedation/general anaesthesia
  - Dorsal position
  - Pulse oximetry/respiratory control
  - Tracheo-/bronchoscopy
  - Lavage catheter: intravenous catheter 45cm 1.4 × 2.1mm

- **Technique**
  - Insert the lavage catheter into the trachea through the biopsy channel until it becomes visible in the bronchus
  - Inject 10–20ml warm saline (0.5–1.0ml/kg)
  - Aspirate immediately (syringe/suction pump)
  - Consider repeating this procedure
  - Remove the lavage catheter
  - Remove the endoscope
  - Consider oxygenation
  - Process the sample

Complications

- Respiratory arrest
- Cough
- Aspiration pneumonia

Endotracheal Lavage (Flexible Endoscope)

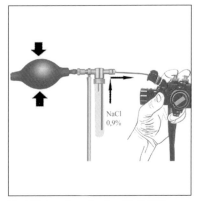

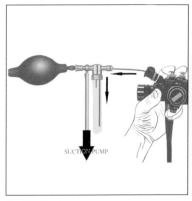

Fig 4.79 Insertion of saline (NaCl 0.9% = physiological saline)

Fig 4.80 Suction

Method

- **Preparation**
  - Sedation/general anaesthesia
  - Dorsal position
  - Pulse oximetry/respiratory control
  - Tracheo-/bronchoscopy
  - Required flushing system: male dog urinary catheter versus aspirator and bronchus flusher system by Storz (as per illustration)

- **Technique**
  - Insert the endoscope into the bronchus
  - Fill a glass tube with 10ml of warm saline
  - Insert the lavage catheter into the trachea through the biopsy channel until it is visible in the bronchus
  - Inject physiological saline by manually pumping the rubber bellow (Storz)
  - Aspirate immediately by using the suction pump
  - Consider repeating the procedure
  - Remove the lavage catheter
  - Remove the endoscope
  - Consider oxygenation
  - Process the sample

Complications

- Respiratory arrest
- Cough
- Aspiration pneumonia

Endotracheal Lavage (Endotracheal Tube)

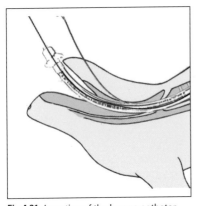

Fig 4.81 Insertion of the lavage catheter into the endotracheal tube

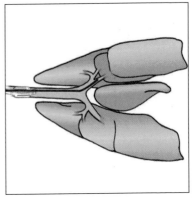

Fig 4.82 Insertion of the lavage catheter into the bronchus

Method

- **Preparation**
  - Sedation/general anaesthesia
  - Dorsal position
  - Pulse oximetry/respiratory control
  - Tracheo-/bronchoscopy
  - Endotracheal intubation

- **Technique**
  - Direct lavage
  - Instil 5–10ml of warm physiological saline directly into the endotracheal tube via a syringe adapter
  - Aspirate immediately
  - Indirect lavage
  - Insert the lavage catheter into the endotracheal tube
  - Continue to feed this into the bronchus
  - Instil 5–10ml of warm physiological saline
  - Aspirate immediately

Complications

- Respiratory arrest
- Cough
- Aspiration pneumonia

Transtracheal Lavage

Indication

- Tracheobronchitis of unknown origin

Transtracheal Lavage

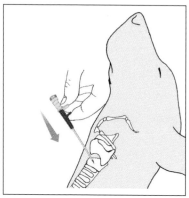

Fig 4.83 Puncture the trachea

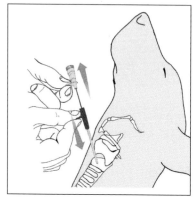

Fig 4.84 Remove the needle

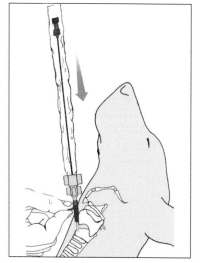

Fig 4.85 Attach and insert a central venous catheter

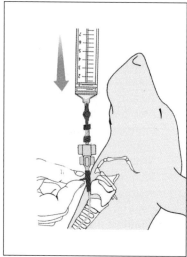

Fig 4.86 Instil some saline

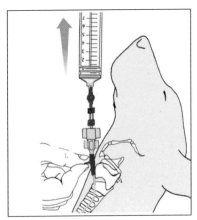

Fig 4.87 Aspirate/remove saline by suction

Method

- **Preparation**
  - Topical anaesthesia, possibly sedation
  - Sitting position with a lifted head and extended neck
  - Clip fur/disinfect skin
  - System: central venous catheter

- **Technique**
  - Puncture the trachea with an over-the-needle catheter between the thyroid and cricoid cartilage or the first two tracheal rings
  - Remove the needle and leave the catheter in place
  - Attach and insert the central venous catheter through to the bifurcation (lavage catheter)
  - Instil 10–20ml of warm saline (0.5–1.0ml/kg)
  - Aspirate immediately with a syringe or suction pump
  - Remove the venous and lavage catheter
  - Process the sample

Complications

- Respiratory arrest
- Cough
- Aspiration pneumonia

Thoracocentesis

Indication

- Thoracic effusion

Thoracocentesis

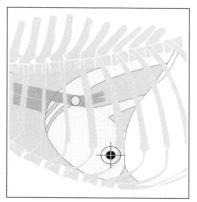

Fig 4.88 Puncture site

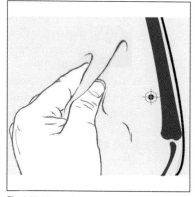

Fig 4.89 Thoracic puncture cranial of the rib

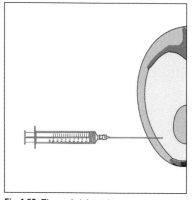

Fig 4.90 Thoracic/pleural puncture

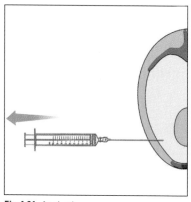

Fig 4.91 Aspiration

Method

- **Preparation**
    - While the patient is standing on the examination table
    - Clip fur/disinfect skin (left/right thoracic wall)
    - Required system: 10ml syringe with a three-way tap and an attached cannula

- **Technique**
    - Puncture site: cranial of the rib in the seventh–eighth intercostal space, dorsal (if pneumothorax), ventral (if pleural effusion)
    - Push the skin towards cranial
    - Puncture the thoracic wall slowly
    - Aspirate air/fluid until a negative pressure has been created
    - Consider closing the three-way tap and changing the syringe, open the three-way tap again and repeat aspiration
    - Remove the puncture cannula while maintaining insertion angle
    - Let go of the skin that was previously moved forwards
    - Compress the puncture site (2–5 min)
    - Examine and process the sample
    - Take control radiographs

Complications

- Thoracic haemorrhage (rib vessels, lung puncture)
- Pneumothorax (lung puncture)
- Subcutaneous emphysema
- Infection

Further Respiratory Examination Methods

- Laboratory investigation
- Computer tomography (CT)
- Angiography
- Pulse-oximetry
- Thoracoscopy
- Thoracotomy

5 Gastrointestinal Examination Methods

Case History

Principal symptoms

- Vomitus/emesis
- Regurgitation
- Diarrhoea
- Inappetence
- Dysphagia
- Polyphagia
- Hypersalivation
- Weight loss
- Faecal impaction
- Abdominal pain/cramps/colic
- Scooting/licking of the anal region
- Tenesmus

Inspection

Indication

- Part of the general examination

Inspection

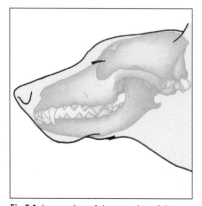

Fig 5.1 Inspection of the muscles of the head

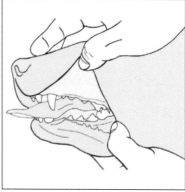

Fig 5.2 Inspection of the teeth

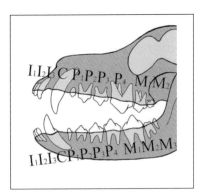

Fig 5.3 Dentition of the dog

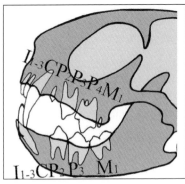

Fig 5.4 Dentition of the cat

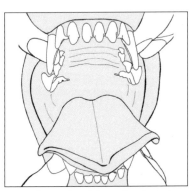

Fig 5.5 Inspection of the oral cavity in the dog

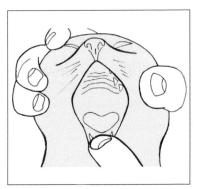

Fig 5.6 Inspection of the oral cavity in the cat

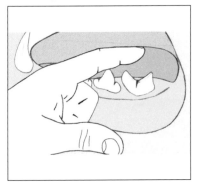

Fig 5.7 Inspection under the tongue

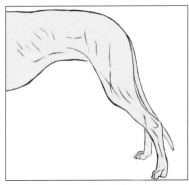

Fig 5.8 Inspection of the abdomen

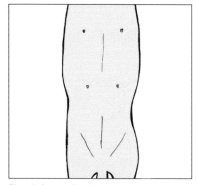

Fig 5.9 Inspection of the abdomen

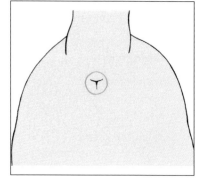

Fig 5.10 Inspection of the perineum and anus

Method

- **Technique**
  - Observe the nutritional status, body posture/stance, muscles of the head, oral cavity, structures of the throat and neck, thorax, abdomen, perineum und anus

- **Evaluation criteria**
  - Size, shape, symmetry, colour

Findings

- **Physiological**
  - Nothing abnormal to detect (NAD)

- **Pathological**

  Nutritional status
  - Cachexia/marasmus
  - Obesity

  Body posture/stance
  - Abdominal pain (praying position, curved back)
  - Tenesmus
  - Increased abdominal girth

  Muscles of the head
  - Muscular atrophy
  - Tetany
  - Tremors

  Oral cavity
  - Facial asymmetry (facial nerve paresis, Horner's syndrome)
  - Lockjaw
  - Cheilitis
  - Underbite/overbite
  - Dental malposition/malocclusion
  - Persistent deciduous teeth (canines)
  - Dental abrasion
  - Dental calculus
  - Paradontitis
  - Tooth decay/resorptive lesions
  - Enamel defect (distemper)
  - Pulpitis
  - Dental fracture
  - Malposition of the jaw (luxation/fracture)
  - Dental fistula (abscess)
  - Papillomatosis
  - Epulis
  - Tumours
  - Gingivitis
  - Stomatitis
  - Tonsillitis/tonsillar tumour
  - Foreign body
  - Glossitis (linear foreign body strangulation)
  - Cleft palate/oronasal fistula
  - Retention cyst of the salivary gland (ranula)

  Structures of the throat/neck
  - Retention cyst of the salivary gland (cyst on the neck/meliceris)
  - Lymph node enlargement (mandibular lymph node)

  Thorax
  - Abdominal respiration

  Abdomen
  - Increased abdominal girth

  Perineum
  - Increased size/bulges/swellings
  - Perianal tumours
  - Perianal fistulas

Palpation

Indication

- Part of the general examination

Palpation: Head/Neck

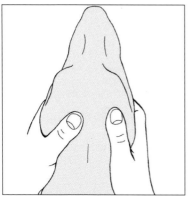

Fig 5.11 Palpation of the muscles of the head

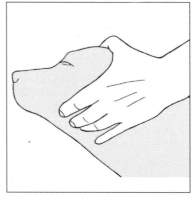

Fig 5.12 Palpation of the muscles of the head

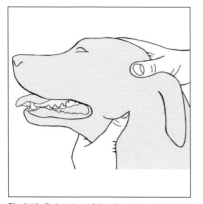

Fig 5.13 Palpation of the throat/neck structures

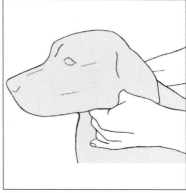

Fig 5.14 Palpation of the salivary glands and mandibular lymph nodes

Palpation: Head

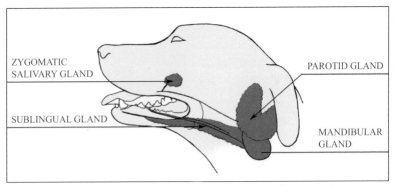

ZYGOMATIC
SALIVARY GLAND

PAROTID GLAND

SUBLINGUAL GLAND

MANDIBULAR
GLAND

Fig 5.15 Salivary glands in the dog (zygomatic salivary gland, sublingual gland, parotid gland, mandibular gland)

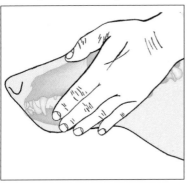

Fig 5.16 Palpation of the lower jaw

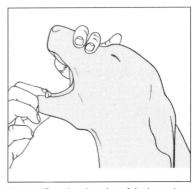

Fig 5.17 Functional testing of the lower jaw

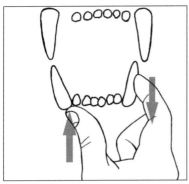

Fig 5.18 Palpation of the lower jaw

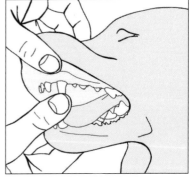

Fig 5.19 Palpation of the teeth

Palpation: Abdomen

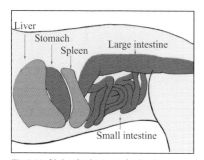

Fig 5.20 Abdominal organs in the dog (left lateral view)

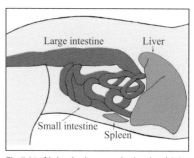

Fig 5.21 Abdominal organs in the dog (right lateral view)

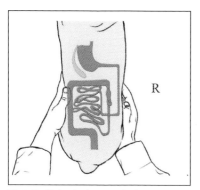

Fig 5.22 Abdominal organs in the dog (dorsal view)

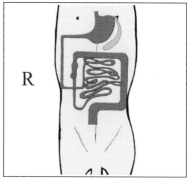

Fig 5.23 Abdominal organs in the dog (ventral view)

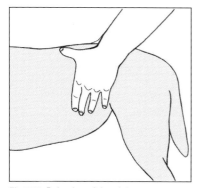

Fig 5.24 Palpation of the abdomen (two hands)

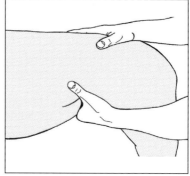

Fig 5.25 Palpation of the abdomen (one hand)

Palpation: Abdomen/Perineum/Rectum

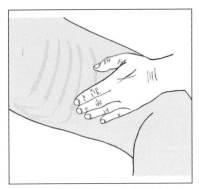

Fig 5.26 Palpation of the cranial abdomen

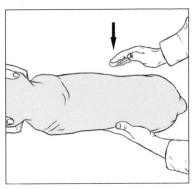

Fig 5.27 Fluid thrill

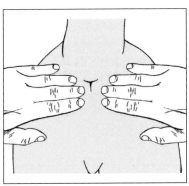

Fig 5.28 Palpation of the perineum

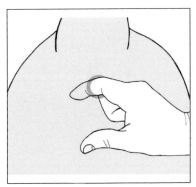

Fig 5.29 Rectal examination of the perineum

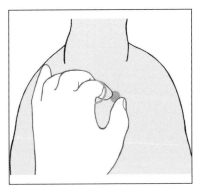

Fig 5.30 Rectal examination of the anal sacs

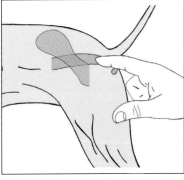

Fig 5.31 Rectal examination

Method

- **Preparation**
    - Usually while the patient is standing on the examination table
    - Possibly in lateral recumbency
    - Possibly while standing on the floor

- **Technique**
    - Palpation of the skull, oral cavity, throat and neck structures, thorax, abdomen, perineum and rectum

- **Evaluation criteria**
    - Size, shape, symmetry, consistency, temperature, painfulness

Findings

- **Physiological**
    - Nothing abnormal to detect (NAD)

- **Pathological**

    Skull
    - Muscle atrophy of the head muscles
    - Luxation/fracture of the jaw
    - Craniomandibular osteopathy (CMO)
    - Osteodystrophia fibrosa (hyperparathyroidism)

    Oral cavity
    - Retention cyst of the sublingual salivary gland (ranula)
    - Tumour
    - Loose/painful teeth

    Throat and neck structures
    - Retention cyst of the sublingual salivary gland (cyst on the throat/meliceris)
    - Lymphadenopathy (mandibular lymph node)

    Thorax
    - Rib fractures
    - Intercostal muscle rupture

Abdomen
- Increased abdominal tension (abdominal pain/acute abdomen)
- Pain on palpation of the cranial abdomen (suspect acute pancreatitis)
- Abdominal effusion (fluid thrill)
- Hernia (umbilical, inguinal, scrotal)
- Organomegaly (liver, spleen, stomach)
- Increased size (intestine, liver, lymph node)
- Faecal impaction

Perineum
- Hernia (perineal hernia)
- Increased size/bulges/swellings (anal sac impaction/abscess/tumour)
- Perianal tumours

Rectum
- Perineal hernia/rectal diverticulum
- Anal sac impaction/abscess/tumour
- Rectal stricture
- Tumour
- Foreign body
- Lymphadenopathy (medial iliac lymph nodes)

Complications

- Painfulness

Percussion

Indication

- Suspected gastric dilation/volvulus in the dog

Percussion

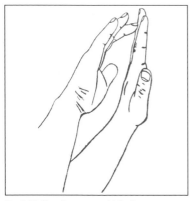

Fig 5.32 Forefinger on middle finger percussion

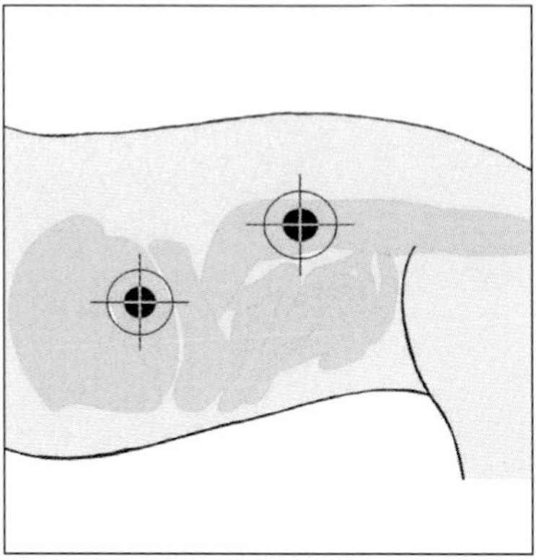

Fig 5.33 Percussion areas

Method

- **Technique**
  - Tap against the lateral abdominal wall (forefinger on middle finger percussion)

Findings

- **Physiological**
  - Subtympanic sound

- **Pathological**
  - Tympanic sound (gastric dilation/volvulus)

Auscultation

Indication

- Part of the general examination

Auscultation

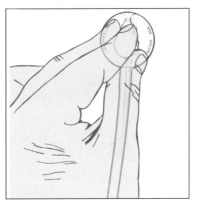

Fig 5.34 Auscultation with a stethoscope

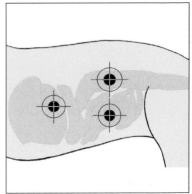

Fig 5.35 Auscultation areas

Method

- **Technique**
  - Listen to the lateral abdominal wall with a stethoscope

Findings

- **Physiological**
  - Nothing abnormal to detect (NAD)

- **Pathological**
  - Hyperperistalsis
  - Hypoperistalsis
  - Complete lack of intestinal sounds (suspected ileus/
    intestinal atony)

Plain X-Ray Study

Indication

- Gastrointestinal disease

X-Ray Study: Plain Study

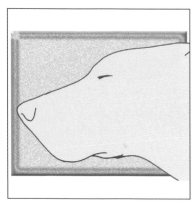

Fig 5.36 Head (lateral view)

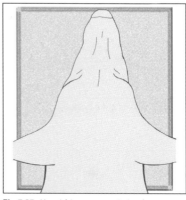

Fig 5.37 Head (dorsoventral view)

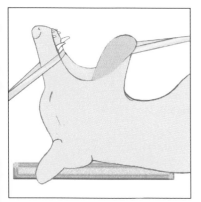

Fig 5.38 Head (rostrocaudal/bullar view)

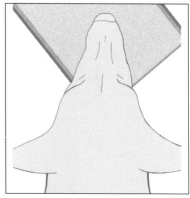

Fig 5.39 Maxilla (intraoral plate)

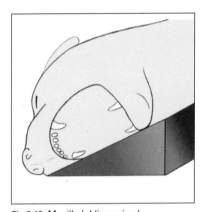

Fig 5.40 Maxilla (oblique view)

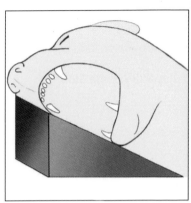

Fig 5.41 Mandible (oblique view)

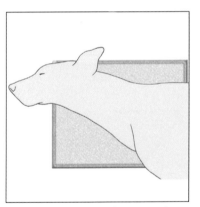

Fig 5.42 Throat and neck (lateral view)

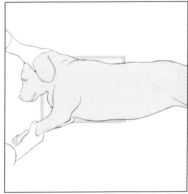

Fig 5.43 Thorax (lateral view)

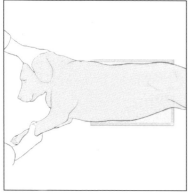

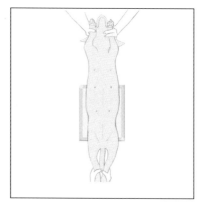

Fig 5.44 Abdomen (lateral view)

Fig 5.45 Abdomen (ventrodorsal view)

Method

- **Technique**
  - Perform a risk/benefit assessment (if the patient is dyspnoeic)
  - Plan and agree the proposed procedure with colleagues and owners
  - Fully inform the owner (consider questions regarding pregnancy and age range)
  - Handle the patient calmly and in a coordinated manner
  - Consider distracting the patient
  - Take two views if at all possible

X-Ray Findings

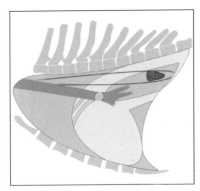

Fig 5.46 Oesophageal foreign body

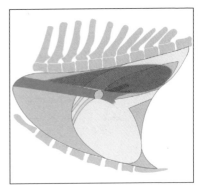

Fig 5.47 Megaoesophagus

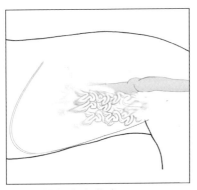

Fig 5.48 Abdominal effusion

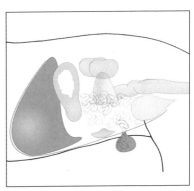

Fig 5.49 (Umbilical) hernia

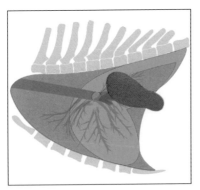

Fig 5.50 Hiatus hernia

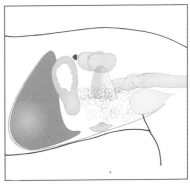

Fig 5.51 Adrenal carcinoma in the dog

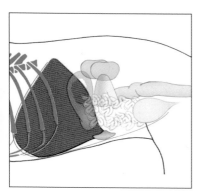

Fig 5.52 Hepatomegaly

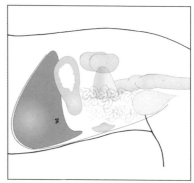

Fig 5.53 Gall bladder stones

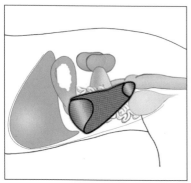

Fig 5.54 Splenic torsion

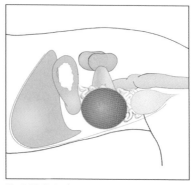

Fig 5.55 Splenic tumour

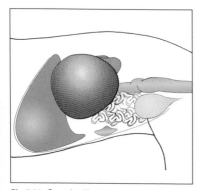

Fig 5.56 Gastric dilation

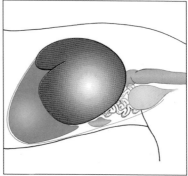

Fig 5.57 Gastric volvulus

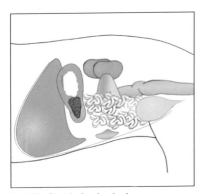

Fig 5.58 Gastric foreign body

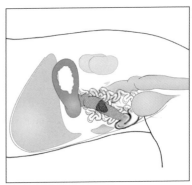

Fig 5.59 Small intestinal foreign body

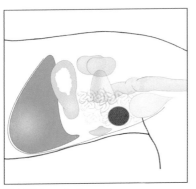

Fig 5.60 Intestinal tumour

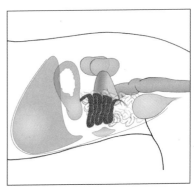

Fig 5.61 Linear foreign body with plication of the intestines

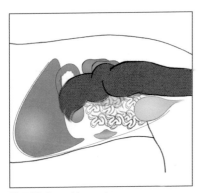

Fig 5.62 Faecal impaction

Findings

- **Physiological**
  - Nothing abnormal to detect (NAD)

- **Pathological**

  Oropharynx
  - Foreign body
  - Tumour
  - Lower or upper jaw fracture/luxation
  - Craniomandibular osteopathy (CMO) (West-Highland White Terrier)
  - Osteodystrophia fibrosa (renal hyperparathyroidism)

  Oesophagus
  - Foreign body
  - Tumour
  - Megaoesophagus
  - Oesophageal stricture
  - Oesophageal rupture

  Abdomen
  - Foreign body
  - Tumour
  - Abdominal effusion
  - Pneumoabdomen
  - Diaphragmatic hernia, hiatus hernia, umbilical hernia, inguinal hernia, scrotal hernia, perineal hernia
  - Adrenal carcinoma

  Liver
  - Hepatomegaly
  - Tumour
  - Calcification
  - Gall bladder stones

  Spleen
  - Splenomegaly
  - Splenic torsion
  - Splenic tumour

Stomach
- Gastric dilation
- Gastric torsion
- Pyloric stenosis
- Tumour
- Foreign body
- Gastric rupture

Small intestine
- Foreign body
- Tumour
- Ileus
- Invagination
- Intestinal rupture
- Volvulus

Large intestine
- Foreign body
- Tumour
- Faecal impaction
- Megacolon
- Invagination (caecum)
- Perineal hernia

Complications

- Traumatic injury on the X-ray table
- Respiratory arrest (dyspnoea)
- Radiation exposure
- Aspiration pneumonia (in case of contrast medium application)
- Peritonitis (barium sulphate application in case of gastrointestinal perforation)

Gastrointestinal Contrast Medium Study

Indication

- Inconclusive result after plain radiography of the gastrointestinal tract
- Suspected foreign body

Gastrointestinal Contrast Medium Study

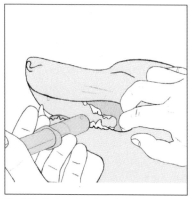

Fig 5.63 Oral application of the contrast medium

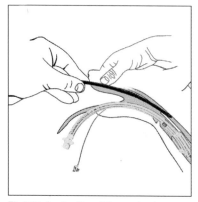

Fig 5.64 Application of the contrast medium via a gastric tube

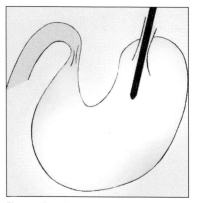

Fig 5.65 Position of the gastric tube

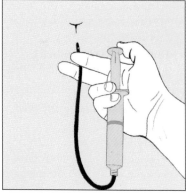

Fig 5.66 Rectal application of the contrast medium

Method (Gastrointestinal Contrast Medium Study)

- **Barium Sulphate (80–100 per cent)**

  Indication
  - Suspected ileus, foreign body, tumours, pyloric stenosis, hernias, motility disorders
  - Contraindication: suspected gastrointestinal perforation

  Oral application
  - 7–12ml/kg

  Gastric tube
  - Sedation
  - Endotracheal intubation and cuffing of the tube
  - Right lateral recumbency
  - Mark the required length of the gastric tube (oral cavity – stomach)
  - Moisten the gastric tube with water and insert it over the endotracheal tube
  - Listen to the sound coming through the gastric tube (stomach or respiratory sounds)
  - Instil 5–10ml saline (discontinue if the patient coughs)
  - Apply the contrast medium 4–8ml/kg
  - Fold over the end of the gastric tube and pull it out

  X-ray views
  - Right lateral + ventrodorsal
  - Take radiographs of the dog immediately and after 15/30/60/90 min
  - Take radiographs of the cat immediately and after 15/30/45/60/90 min

- **Iodine (Gastrografin®)**

  Indication
  - Suspected gastrointestinal perforation

  Oral application/gastric tube
  - 2–3ml/kg

  X-ray views
  - Right lateral + ventrodorsal
  - Take radiographs immediately and after 15/30/45/60/90 min

- **Double-contrast gastrography**

  Indication
  - Mucosal detail, foreign body, tumour

Gastric tube
- Application of barium sulphate 1–2ml/kg
- Application of air 10–20ml/kg (achieves slight gastric expansion)

X-ray views
- Right lateral + ventrodorsal
- Take radiographs immediately and after 15/30 min
- Remove the air (gastric tube/gastric compression)

Method (Swallow Study)

- **Barium Sulphate (30 per cent)**
  - Mix the barium sulphate-suspension with a tin of dog food
  - Perform a video recording of the food ingestion via fluoroscopy (C-arch)

Method (Colonic Contrast Medium Study)

- **Barium Sulphate (80–100 per cent)**

  ### Indication
  - Suspected stricture, ulcer, tumour, megacolon, perineal hernia

  ### Preparation
  - Fasting period of 12–24 hours
  - Rectal evacuation (saline enema about 6 hours prior to the contrast medium study)

  ### Rectal tube
  - Lubricate a gastric tube
  - Insert the tube gently (2–4cm)
  - Apply the contrast medium: 10–15 ml/kg barium sulphate

  ### X-ray views
  - Right lateral + ventrodorsal
  - Take radiographs immediately and possibly after 15 min

- **Double-contrast colography**

  ### Indication
  - Suspected ulcer, tumour

  ### Rectal tube
  - Lubricate a gastric tube
  - Insert the tube gently (2–4cm)
  - Apply the contrast medium: 10–15ml/kg barium sulphate
  - Allow the contrast medium to run out
  - Instil about 5ml/kg of air

  ### X-ray views
  - Right lateral + ventrodorsal
  - Take radiographs immediately and possibly after 15 min

Endoscopy: Gastroscopy

Indication

- Further diagnostic investigation into gastrointestinal disease of unknown origin
- Melaena, chronic vomiting, haematemesis, chronic small intestinal diarrhoea, pain

Gastroscopy

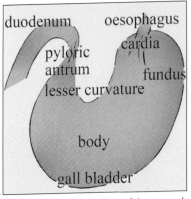

Fig 5.67 Anatomical regions of the stomach

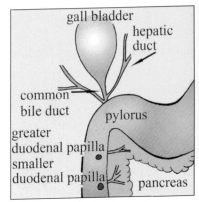

Fig 5.68 Anatomical regions of the duodenum

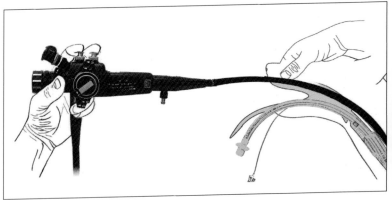

Fig 5.69 Insertion of the flexible endoscope

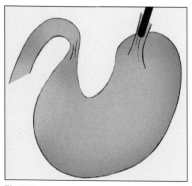

Fig 5.70 Gastroscopy (step 1, oesophagus and cardia)

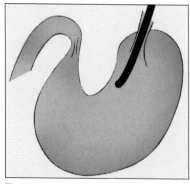

Fig 5.71 Gastroscopy (step 2, lesser curvature)

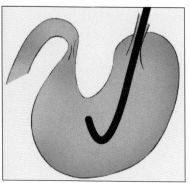

Fig 5.72 Gastroscopy (step 3, angular notch)

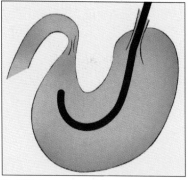

Fig 5.73 Gastroscopy (step 4, pyloric antrum)

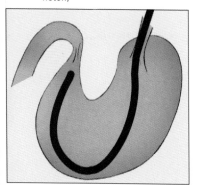

Fig 5.74 Gastroscopy (step 5, pylorus)

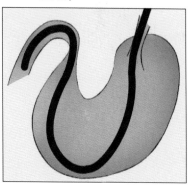

Fig 5.75 Gastroscopy (step 6, duodenum)

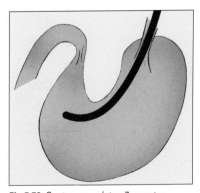

Fig 5.76 Gastroscopy (step 7, greater curvature/body)

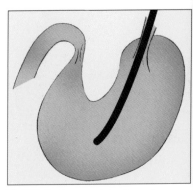

Fig 5.77 Gastroscopy (step 8, greater curvature/body)

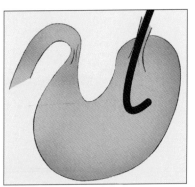

Fig 5.78 Gastroscopy (step 9, fundus)

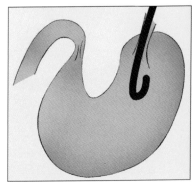

Fig 5.79 Gastroscopy (step 10, cardia)

Method

- **Preparation**
  - Sedation/general anaesthesia
  - Laryngoscopy
  - Endotracheal intubation
  - Left lateral recumbency

- **Technique**
  - Insert the fibre endoscope gently under visual control and air insufflation
  - Suction off the air after the procedure

- **Order**
  - Oesophagus
  - Cardia
  - Lesser curvature
  - Angular notch
  - Pyloric antrum
  - Pylorus
  - Duodenum
  - Greater curvature/body
  - Fundus
  - Cardia (retroflexion)
  - Oesophagus

Findings

- **Physiological**
  - Nothing abnormal to detect (NAD)
- **Pathological**
  - Haemorrhage
  - Foreign body
  - Gastritis ± ulcer/erosion
  - Tumour
  - Stricture
  - Pyloric stenosis
  - Gastric dilation
  - Diverticulum
  - Hiatus hernia

Complications

- Haemorrhages
- Stomach perforation

Coloscopy

Indication

- Further diagnostic investigation into large intestinal disease of unknown origin

Coloscopy

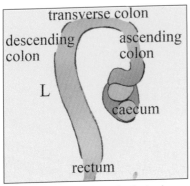

Fig 5.80 Anatomy of the colon in the dog

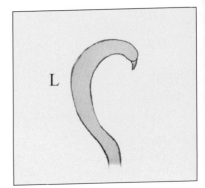

Fig 5.81 Colon in the cat

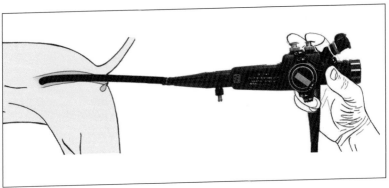

Fig 5.82 Insertion of the endoscope

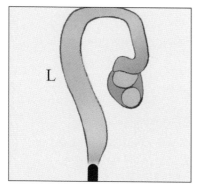

Fig 5.83 Coloscopy (step 1, rectum)

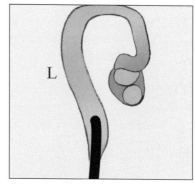

Fig 5.84 Coloscopy (step 2, descending colon)

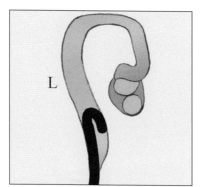

Fig 5.85 Coloscopy (step 3, rectum)

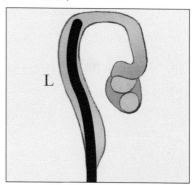

Fig 5.86 Coloscopy (step 4, descending colon)

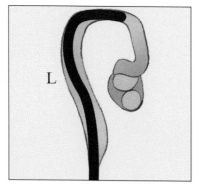

Fig 5.87 Coloscopy (step 5, transverse colon)

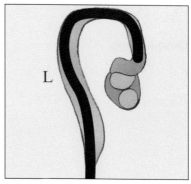

Fig 5.88 Coloscopy (step 6, ascending colon)

Method (Coloscopy)

- **Preparation**
  - Fasting period of 12–24 hours
  - Rectal evacuation (saline enema about 6 hours prior to the coloscopy)
  - Sedation/general anaesthesia
  - Left lateral recumbency

- **Technique**
  - Lubricate the fibre endoscope
  - Gently insert the fibre endoscope under visual control and air insufflation
  - Suction off the air at the end of the procedure

- **Order**
  - Rectum
  - Retroflexion
  - Descending colon
  - Transverse colon
  - Ascending colon (caecum/ileocaecal opening)

- **Physiological**
  - Nothing abnormal to detect (NAD)

- **Pathological**
  - Haemorrhage
  - Foreign body
  - Colitis ± ulcer/erosion
  - Tumour
  - Stricture
  - Megacolon

Complications

- Faecal matter in the rectum
- Haemorrhage
- Colon perforation

Ultrasound Examination: Abdomen

Indication

- Further diagnostic investigation of organ disease, tumours

Ultrasound Examination

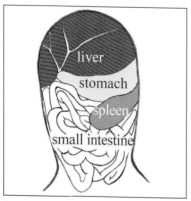

Fig 5.89 Position of the cranial abdominal organs

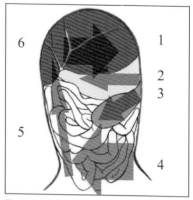

Fig 5.90 Order of the ultrasound examination

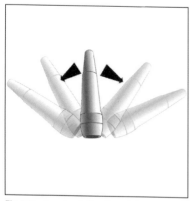

Fig 5.91 Angular deflection of the probe

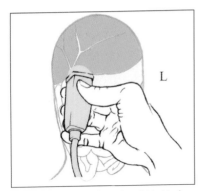

Fig 5.92 Ultrasound (step 1, gall bladder)

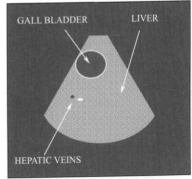

Fig 5.93 Ultrasound image (gall bladder)

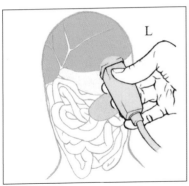

Fig 5.94 Ultrasound (step 2, liver)

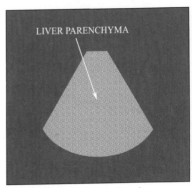

Fig 5.95 Ultrasound image (liver)

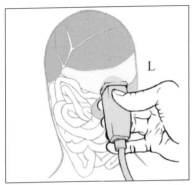

Fig 5.96 Ultrasound (step 3, stomach wall)

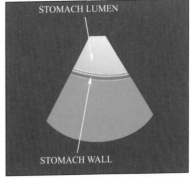

Fig 5.97 Ultrasound image (stomach wall)

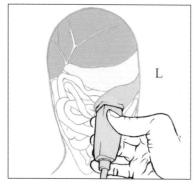

Fig 5.98 Ultrasound (step 4, spleen)

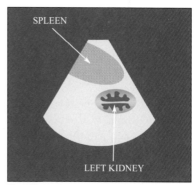

Fig 5.99 Ultrasound image (spleen)

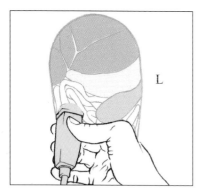

Fig 5.100 Ultrasound (step 5, intestines)

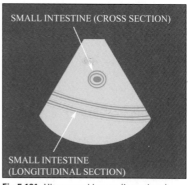

Fig 5.101 Ultrasound image (intestines)

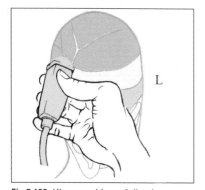

Fig 5.102 Ultrasound (step 6, liver)

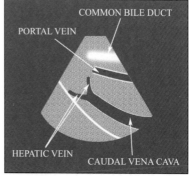

Fig 5.103 Ultrasound image (liver)

Method

- **Preparation**
  - Dorsal position
  - Clip fur as necessary
  - Ultrasound gel
  - Sector/linear transducer 7.5 MHz

- **Technique**
  - Place the probe median, paramedian or transverse to the abdominal wall caudal of the costal arch
  - Turn and pan the transducer in all directions

- **Order**
  - Liver
  - Stomach
  - Spleen
  - Intestines
  - Liver

Findings

- **Physiological**
  - Nothing abnormal to detect (NAD)

- **Pathological**

  Liver
  - Hepatic lipidosis
  - Hepatic congestion
  - Hepatic cirrhosis
  - Tumour
  - Abscess
  - Cyst
  - Possibly portosystemic shunt
  - Portal vein thrombosis

  Gall bladder/bile ducts
  - Cholecystitis
  - Cholelithiasis (gall bladder stones)
  - Tumour/polyp

  Stomach
  - Foreign body
  - Tumour
  - Hyperperistalsis/atony
  - Possibly stomach rupture

Lymph Node Biopsy

Indication

- Lymphadenopathy

Lymph Node Biopsy

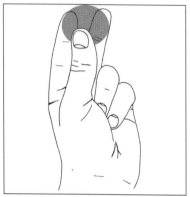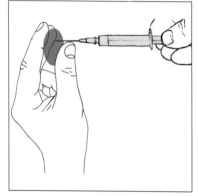

Fig 5.104 Fixation of the lymph node

Fig 5.105 Fine needle aspiration of the lymph node

Method

- **Preparation**
  - Clip fur
  - Disinfect skin

- **Technique**
  - Fixate the lymph node between your thumb, fore and middle finger
  - Puncture the lymph node with a hypodermic needle and an attached syringe
  - Aspirate
  - Remove the hypodermic needle/syringe
  - Compress the puncture site with a swab
  - Smear the sample onto a microscope slide

Complications

- Painfulness
- Haemorrhage

Tumour biopsy

Indication

- Mass of unknown origin

Tumour Biopsy

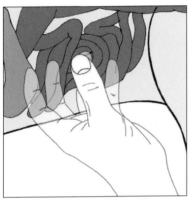

Fig 5.106 Fixation of the tumour

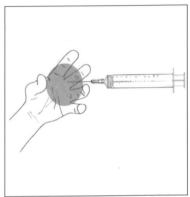

Fig 5.107 Puncture and aspiration of the tumour

Method

- **Preparation**
  - Clip fur
  - Disinfect skin

- **Technique**
  - Fixate the tumour manually
  - Gently puncture the tumour with a hypodermic needle and an attached syringe through the lateral abdominal wall
  - Aspirate
  - Remove the hypodermic needle/syringe
  - Compress the puncture site with a swab
  - Smear the sample onto a microscope slide

Complications

- Painfulness
- Haemorrhage
- Metastasis

Liver Biopsy

Indication

- Liver disease of unknown origin

Liver Biopsy

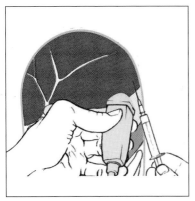

Fig 5.108 Fine needle liver biopsy

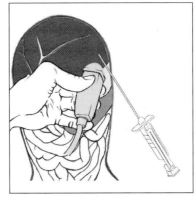

Fig 5.109 Tru-cut liver biopsy

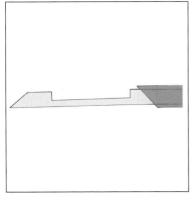

Fig 5.110 Tru-cut-type biopsy needle
(step 1)

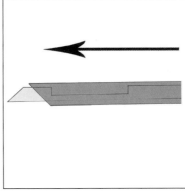

Fig 5.111 Tru-cut-type biopsy needle
(step 2)

Method

- **Preparation**
  - Blood laboratory analysis including coagulation status
  - Dorsal position (possibly sedation)
  - Clip fur/disinfect skin

- **Technique**
  - Ultrasound examination
  - Puncture the liver tangential to the ultrasound probe under the costal arch while using ultrasound control
  - Aspirate and remove the hypodermic needle/syringe during the aspiration process or release the punch mechanism (Tru-cut biopsy)
  - Smear the sample onto a microscope slide or place it into a fixation solution (Tru-cut biopsy)

Complications

- Pneumothorax
- Haemorrhages

Gastric/Intestinal Biopsy

Indication

- Gastroenteritis of unknown origin

Gastric/Intestinal Biopsy

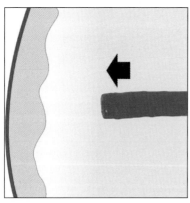

Fig 5.112 Endoscopic localisation of the biopsy site

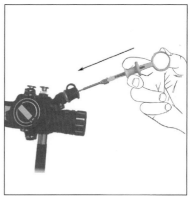

Fig 5.113 Insertion of the biopsy forceps

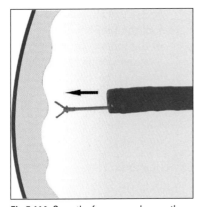

Fig 5.114 Open the forceps and grasp the mucosa

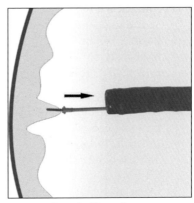

Fig 5.115 Close the biopsy forceps

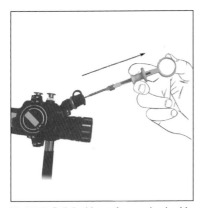

Fig 5.116 Pull the biopsy forceps back with a sudden jerk

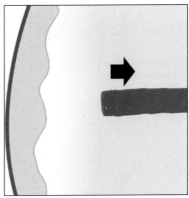

Fig 5.117 Check the biopsy site

Method

- **Preparation**
  - Sedation
  - Possibly endotracheal intubation
  - Endoscopic pre-examination

- **Technique**
  - Localize the biopsy site with the endoscope
  - Insert the biopsy forceps into the biopsy channel of the fibre endoscope
  - Open the biopsy forceps
  - Grasp the mucosa
  - Close the biopsy forceps
  - Pull the biopsy forceps back with a sudden jerk
  - Pull the biopsy forceps out of the biopsy channel
  - Transfer the biopsy sample into fixation solution with the help of a sterile hypodermic needle
  - Check the biopsy site with the endoscope

Complications

- Haemorrhage
- Gastric/intestinal perforation

Rectal Swab Sample

Indication

- Rectal disease of unknown origin

Rectal Swab Sample

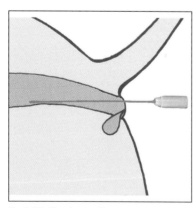

Fig 5.118 Swab sampling

Method

- **Technique**
  - Insert the swab into the rectum
  - Swab the mucosa
  - Smear the sample onto a microscope slide

Complications

- Haemorrhage

Abdominocentesis

Indication

- Abdominal effusion

Abdominocentesis

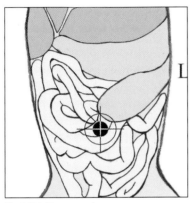

Fig 5.119 Puncture site

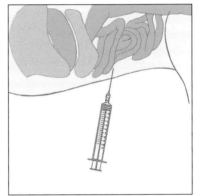

Fig 5.120 Abdominal puncture

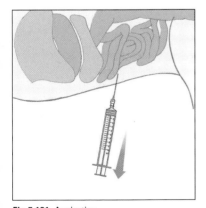

Fig 5.121 Aspiration

Method

- **Preparation**
  - Lateral recumbency
  - Clip fur and disinfect skin

- **Technique**
  - Possible evacuation of the urinary bladder required
  - Puncture the abdominal wall paramedian and caudal of the umbilicus with syringe and attached hypodermic needle
  - Direct the puncture needle towards caudal
  - Aspirate
  - Remove the syringe and needle

Complications

- Splenic puncture
- Intestinal puncture
- Puncture of the urinary bladder
- Peritonitis

Further Gastrointestinal Examination Methods

- **Laboratory investigations**
  - Blood
  - Faeces

- **Laparoscopy**
  - Laparotomy
  - Cholecystocentesis
  - Endoscopic retrograde cholangiopancreaticography (ERCP)

6 Urological Examination Methods

Case History

Principal Symptoms

- Polydipsia
- Polyuria
- Oliguria/anuria
- Vomitus
- Stranguria
- Pollakisuria
- Haematuria
- Halitosis
- Anorexia/inappetence
- Urinary incontinence
- Urinary retention

Inspection

Indication

- Part of the general examination

Method

- **Technique**
  - Observe the body posture/stance, body condition and respiration at rest
  - Look at the oral mucous membranes
  - Look at the vulva/penis
  - Look at the coat/fur

Findings

- **Physiological**
  - Costoabdominal respiration/respiratory rate 10–30/min
  - Pink mucous membrane colour

- **Pathological**
  - Oral mucous membranes
  - Pallor (anaemia)
  - Ulcer

Palpation

Indication

- Part of the general examination

Palpation

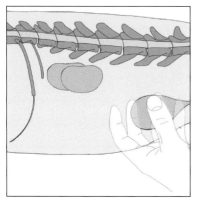

Fig 6.1 Palpation of the urinary bladder

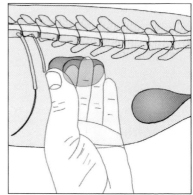

Fig 6.2 Palpation of the kidneys in the cat

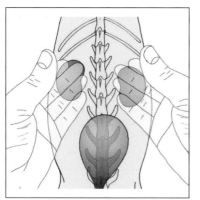

Fig 6.3 Palpation of the kidneys in the dog and cat

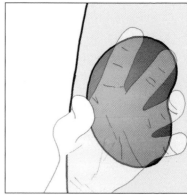

Fig 6.4 Palpation of the right kidney

Method

- **Technique**

  Urinary bladder
  - Feel the bladder

  Kidneys
  - Feel the kidneys and compare them with each other

- **Evaluation criteria**
  - Size, shape, symmetry, position, consistency

Findings

- **Physiological**

  Urinary bladder
  - The size depends on the fullness of the bladder
  - Soft and fluctuating consistency

  Kidneys
  - The right kidney lies further cranial than the left one; they should feel symmetric and be of semi-firm consistency

- **Pathological**

  Urinary bladder
  - Taut/distended full bladder (urinary obstruction, spinal lesion)

  Kidneys
  - Renomegaly (uni-/bilateral)
  - Decreased kidney size (uni-/bilateral)
  - Softer consistency than expected (acute renal failure)
  - More solid consistency than expected (chronic renal failure)
  - Painfulness (retroperitoneal haemorrhage/haematoma/abscess, peritonitis, ureteral obstruction)

Plain X-Ray Study

Indication

- Renal and urinary tract disease

X-Ray Study: Plain Study

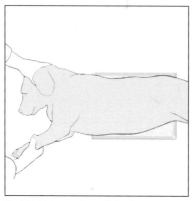

Fig 6.5 Abdomen (lateral view)

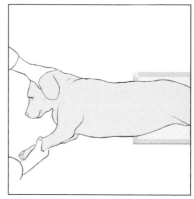

Fig 6.6 Pelvis (lateral view)

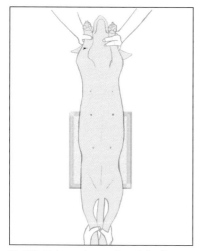

Fig 6.7 Abdomen (ventrodorsal view)

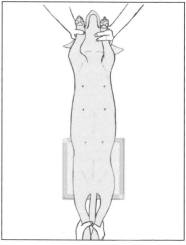

Fig 6.8 Pelvis (ventrodorsal view)

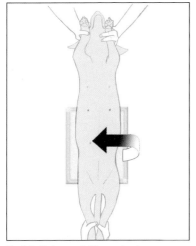

Fig 6.9 Abdomen (oblique view)

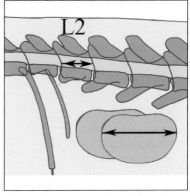

Fig 6.10 Measurement of the kidney size

Method

- **Technique**
    - Perform a risk/benefit assessment (if the patient is dyspnoeic)
    - Plan and agree the proposed procedure with colleagues and owners
    - Fully inform the owner (consider questions about pregnancy and age range)
    - Hande the patient calmly and in a coordinated manner
    - Consider distracting the patient
    - Take two views if at all possible
    - Oblique view for visualisation of the ureters (excretory urography)

X-Ray Findings

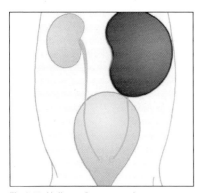

Fig 6.11 Unilateral renomegaly

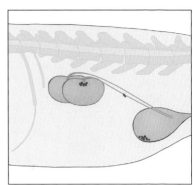

Fig 6.12 Calculi in the kidney, urethra and bladder

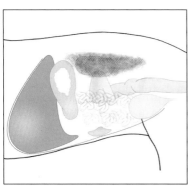

Fig 6.13 Retroperitoneal haematoma

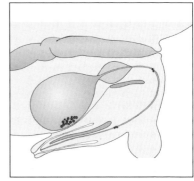

Fig 6.14 Calculi in the male dog

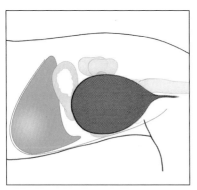

Fig 6.15 Atony of the urinary bladder

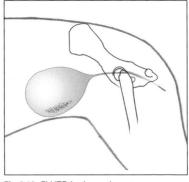

Fig 6.16 FLUTD in the male cat

Findings

- **Physiological**

Kidneys
- Position: the right kidney lies further cranial than the left one
- Size in the dog: 2.5–3.5 × length of the second lumbar vertebra (L2)
- Size in the cat: 2.5–3.0 × length of the second lumbar vertebra (L2)

- **Pathological**

Kidneys
- Uni-/bilateral renomegaly
- Decreased size of the kidneys
- Calculi
- Renal haemorrhage/retroperitoneal haematoma

Ureters
- Calculi

Urinary bladder
- Calculi
- Emphysematous cystitis
- Atony of the urinary bladder
- FLUTD in the male cat

Urethra
- Calculi
- Urethral rupture (urethrography)
- Urethral stricture (urethrography)

Contrast Medium Study

Indication

- Suspected ectopic ureters
- Suspected urachal cyst

X-Ray Study: Excretory Urography

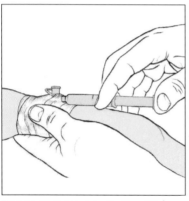

Fig 6.17 Intravenous application of the contrast medium

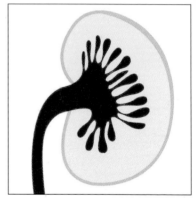

Fig 6.18 Visualisation of the renal pelvis

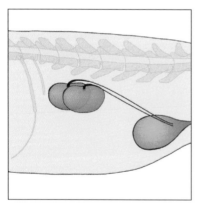

Fig 6.19 Visualisation of the ureters (lateral view)

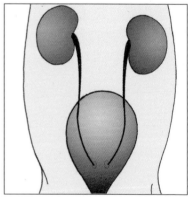

Fig 6.20 Visualisation of the ureters (ventrodorsal view)

X-Ray Study: Cystography

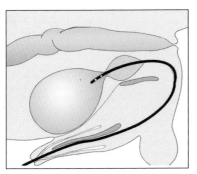

Fig 6.21 Contrast medium application via urinary catheter (male)

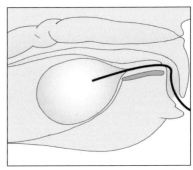

Fig 6.22 Contrast medium application via urinary catheter (female)

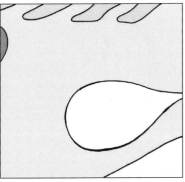

Fig 6.23 Positive contrast cystography (Urografin®)

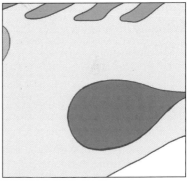

Fig 6.24 Negative contrast cystography (air)

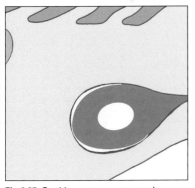

Fig 6.25 Double contrast cystography

X-Ray Study: Urethrography

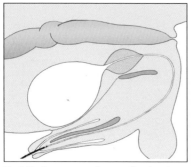 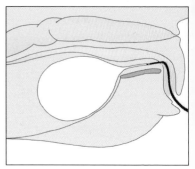

Fig 6.26 Contrast medium application via urinary catheter (male)

Fig 6.27 Contrast medium application via urinary catheter (female)

Excretory Urography

- **Technique**
  - Indication: visualisation of the renal pelvis and the course of the ureters
  - Fasting (12 hours)
  - Enema (1–2 hours prior to procedure)
  - Intravenous catheter placement
  - Intravenous application of the contrast medium: iodine (Urografin®) 400 mg/kg as bolus
  - X-ray views: take the radiographs immediately (ventrodorsal view), after 5 min (ventrodorsal, lateral and oblique view), after 20 min (ventrodorsal view) and possibly after 40 min

Cystography

- **Technique**
  - Indication: visualisation of detail in the urinary bladder
  - Fasting (12 hours)
  - Enema (1 hour prior to the procedure)
  - Urinary catheter placement and evacuation of the bladder
  - Dilute the contrast medium with physiological saline to 100–150mg/ml iodine (Urografin®)
  - Apply the contrast medium:

Positive contrast
- Iodine (Urografin®): c. 10–40ml (cat), 40–200ml (dog)

Negative contrast
- Air: c. 10–40ml (cat), 40–200ml (dog)

Double contrast
1. Iodine (Urografin®): c. 10–40ml
2. Massage the urinary bladder for even distribution
3. Air: c. 10–40ml (cat), 40–200ml (dog)
4. X-ray views: take radiographs immediately (lateral, possibly ventrodorsal view)

Urethrography

- **Technique**
  - Indication: visualisation of the urethra
  - Insert the urinary catheter into the proximal aspect of the urethra
  - Dilute the contrast medium with saline to 100–150mg/ml iodine (Urografin®)
  - Apply the contrast medium:

    Positive contrast
    - Iodine (Urografin®): c. 5–10ml by slow application
    - X-ray views: while the contrast medium is being applied (lateral view, possibly oblique view)

Endoscopy: Urethro-/Cystoscopy

Indication

- Urinary tract disease in the female dog and perineal fistula in the male dog
- Inflammation/haemorrhage of unknown origin, biopsy, lithotripsy

Urethro-/Cystoscopy

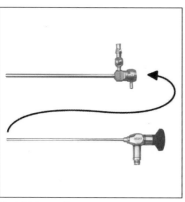

Fig 6.28 Insert the endoscope into the shaft

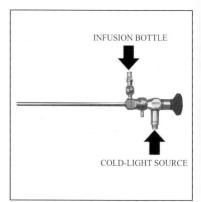

Fig 6.29 Rigid cystoscope (Infusionsflasche = infusion bottle, Kaltlichtquelle = cold-light source)

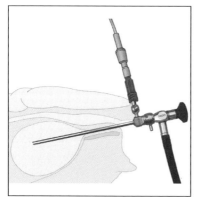

Fig 6.30 Insert the cystoscope into the urethra

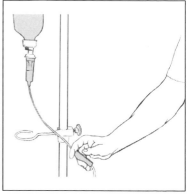

Fig 6.31 Flush the cystoscope

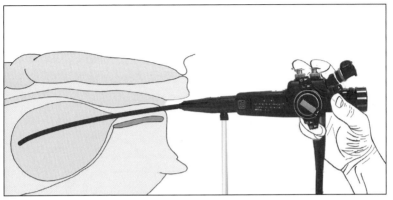

Fig 6.32 Cystoscopy with a flexible endoscope

Method

- **System**
  - Rigid cystoscope 1.9/2.1mm, guide shaft 10 Charr
  - Flexible cystoscope 2.5mm

- **Preparation**
  - Sedation/general anaesthesia

  Rigid cystoscope
  - Insert the endoscope into the shaft
  - Attach an infusion bottle (physiological saline)

  Flexible cystoscope
  - Attach an infusion bottle to the flushing port

- **Technique**
  - Insert the endoscope into the urethra under visual control

- **Order**
  - Vulva–urethra–urinary bladder–ureteral opening

Findings

- **Physiological**
  - Nothing abnormal to detect (NAD)

- **Pathological**
  - Cystitis
  - Tumour/polyp
  - Ruptured urinary bladder or urethra
  - Calculi
  - Ectopic ureters
  - Urachal cyst
  - Localisation of haemorrhage (e.g., renal haemorrhage)

Ultrasound Examination

Indication

- Urinary tract disease of unknown origin

Ultrasound Examination: Urinary Bladder

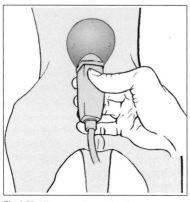

Fig 6.33 Ultrasound examination (transverse axis)

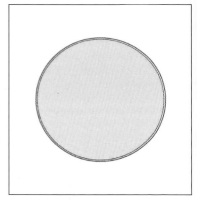

Fig 6.34 Ultrasonic pattern of the urinary bladder in the transverse axis

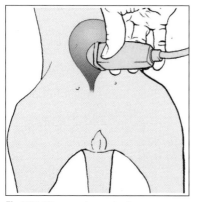

Fig 6.35 Ultrasound examination (longitudinal axis)

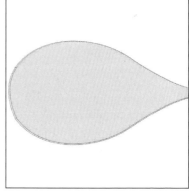

Fig 6.36 Ultrasonic pattern of the urinary bladder in the longitudinal axis

Ultrasound Examination: Kidneys

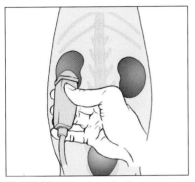

Fig 6.37 Ultrasound examination (transverse axis)

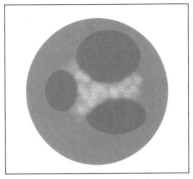

Fig 6.38 Ultrasonic pattern of the kidney in the transverse axis

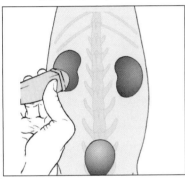

Fig 6.39 Ultrasound examination (longitudinal axis)

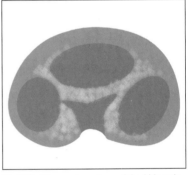

Fig 6.40 Ultrasonic pattern of the kidney in the longitudinal axis

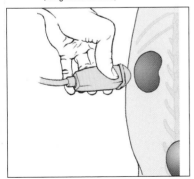

Fig 6.41 Ultrasound examination (longitudinal axis) through the lateral abdominal wall

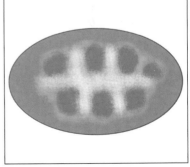

Fig 6.42 Ultrasonic pattern of the kidney in the longitudinal axis

Method

- **Preparation**
  - Dorsal position
  - Clip fur as required
  - Ultrasound gel
  - Sector/linear transducer 5–7.5 MHz

- **Technique**
  - Place the probe perpendicular to the abdomen
  - Turn probe by 90°

- **Order**
  - Left kidney–urinary bladder–right kidney

Findings

- **Physiological**
  - Nothing abnormal to detect (NAD)

- **Pathological**

  Kidneys
  - Retroperitoneal haemorrhage/haematoma/abscess
  - Tumour
  - Calculi
  - Renal cirrhosis
  - Infarction
  - Calcification
  - Cysts (solitary/polycystic)
  - Abscess
  - Hypoplasia/aplasia
  - Hydronephrosis
  - Pyelonephritis

  Ureters
  - Dilation (hydronephrosis)
  - Tumour
  - Calculi

  Urinary bladder
  - Cystitis
  - Tumour
  - Calculi
  - Urachal cyst
  - Rupture

Biopsy of the Urinary Bladder

Indication

• Chronic urinary tract disease of unknown origin

Biopsy of the Urinary Bladder (Rigid Endoscope)

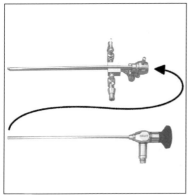

Fig 6.43 Insert the endoscope into the shaft

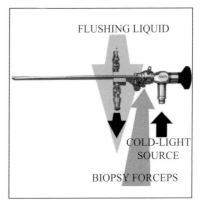

FLUSHING LIQUID

COLD-LIGHT SOURCE

BIOPSY FORCEPS

Fig 6.44 (flushing liquid, cold-light source, biopsy forceps)

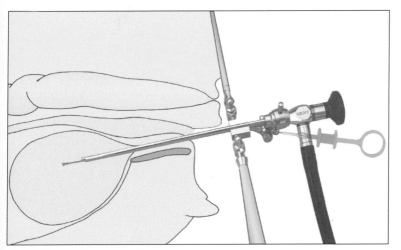

Fig 6.45 Biopsy with a rigid cystoscope

Method

- **System**
  - Cystoscope 1.9/2.1 mm, leading shaft 10 Charr

- **Preparation**
  - General anaesthesia
  - Sternal/prone position
  - Insert the endoscope into the leading shaft
  - Attach the input port with the flushing liquid (infusion bottle with physiological saline)
  - Attach the output port to the flushing liquid (empty infusion bottle)

- **Technique**
  - Insert the endoscope under visual control into the urethra while flushing
  - Localise the biopsy site with the endoscope
  - Insert the biopsy forceps into the leading shaft
  - Open the biopsy forceps
  - Grasp the mucosa
  - Close the biopsy forceps
  - Pull the forceps back with a sudden jerk
  - Pull the biopsy forceps out through the shaft
  - Transfer the sample into a transport medium
  - Check the biopsy site with the endoscope

Complications

- Haemorrhage
- Perforation of the bladder

Biopsy of the Urinary Bladder (Flexible Endoscope)

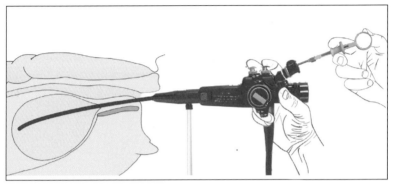

Fig 6.46 Biopsy with a flexible endoscope

Method

- **System**
  - E.g., flexible cystoscope 2.5 mm
- **Preparation**
  - General anaesthesia
  - Sternal/prone position
  - Attach the flushing and suction unit
- **Technique**
  - Insert the endoscope under visual control into the urethra while flushing
  - Localise the biopsy site with the endoscope
  - Insert the biopsy forceps into the leading shaft
  - Open the biopsy forceps
  - Grasp the mucosa
  - Close the biopsy forceps
  - Pull the forceps back with a sudden jerk
  - Pull the biopsy forceps out through the shaft
  - Transfer the sample into a transport medium
  - Check the biopsy site with the endoscope

Complications

- Haemorrhage
- Perforation of the bladder

Biopsy of the Kidney

Indication

• Kidney disease of unknown origin

Biopsy of the Kidney

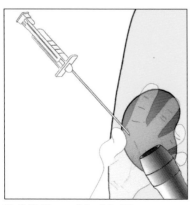

Fig 6.47 Biopsy of the right kidney (dorsal view)

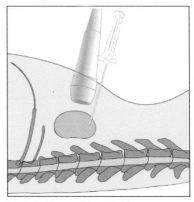

Fig 6.48 Biopsy of the right kidney (lateral view)

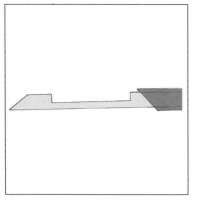

Fig 6.49 Tru-Cut-type biopsy needle (step 1)

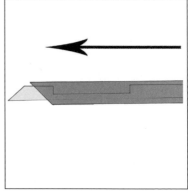

Fig 6.50 Tru-Cut-type biopsy needle (step 2)

Method

- **Preparation**
  - Blood laboratory analysis including coagulation status
  - Dorsal position
  - Sedation/general anaesthesia
  - Clip fur/disinfect skin
  - Ultrasound examination
  - Possibly manual fixation of the kidney

- **Technique**
  - Puncture the renal cortex percutaneously under ultrasound guidance
  - Insert the biopsy needle vertically into the caudal cortical area
  - Release the punch mechanism (Tru-cut biopsy)
  - Remove the biopsy needle
  - Transfer the sample into a transport medium
  - Check the biopsy site via ultrasound (haemorrhage)

Complications

- Haemorrhage
- Infection

Urinary Catheter: Male Dog

Indication

- Urine sample
- Testing for urinary obstruction and sphincter tone in case of spinal disease

Urinary Catheter in the Male Dog

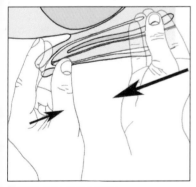

Fig 6.51 Extrude the penis

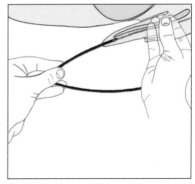

Fig 6.52 Insert the urinary catheter

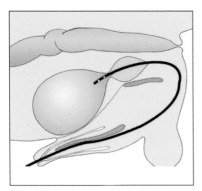

Fig 6.53 Advance the urinary catheter into the bladder

Method

- **Preparation**
  - Standing/lateral recumbency/dorsal position
  - Extrude the penis
  - Possibly clean the penis (in case of balanoposthitis)
  - Measure the required length of the urinary catheter (sterile gloves)
  - Apply sterile lubrication /saline onto the tip of the urinary catheter

- **Technique**
  - Fixate the penis on the penile bone
  - Insert the urinary catheter into the urethra (sterility) until it reaches the bladder neck
  - Catch the urine into a sterile tube
  - Remove the urinary catheter

Complications

- Knotting of the urinary catheter inside the urinary bladder
- Infection
- Perforation of the urethra/bladder

Urinary Catheter: Male Cat

Indication

- Test for urinary obstruction and sphincter tone in case of spinal disease
- Urethral flushing in case of obstruction

Urinary Catheter in the Male Cat

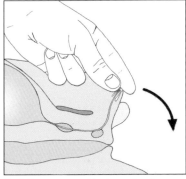

Fig 6.54 Extrude and horizontalise the penis

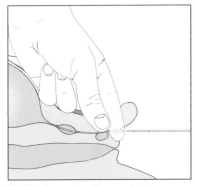

Fig 6.55 Insert the urinary catheter

Method

- **Preparation**
  - Sedation
  - Dorsal position
  - Extrude and horizontalise the penis
  - Apply sterile lubrication gel/saline onto the tip of the urinary catheter

- **Technique**
  - Fixate the penis at the prepuce
  - Insert the urinary catheter into the urethra (sterility) until it reaches the bladder neck, while possibly turning it slightly
  - Catch the urine into a sterile tube
  - Remove the urinary catheter (possibly fixate it via a skin suture in case of urinary obstruction)

Complications

- Perforation of the urethra/urinary bladder
- Infection

Urinary Catheter: Female Dog and Cat

Indication

- Check for urinary obstruction and sphincter tone in case of spinal disease
- Flushing of the urinary bladder

Urinary Catheter in the Female Dog and Cat: Plastic Catheter

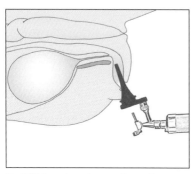

Fig 6.56 Insert an otoscope/speculum vertically

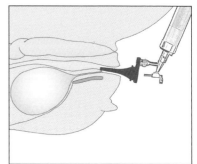

Fig 6.57 Advance the otoscope/speculum horizontally

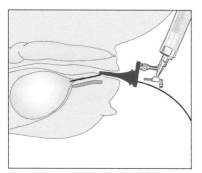

Fig 6.58 Insert the urinary catheter under visual control

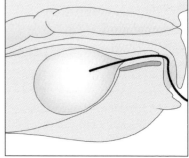

Fig 6.59 Position of the urinary catheter

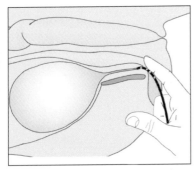

Fig 6.60 Insert the urinary catheter under digital control

Method

- **Preparation**
  - Standing
  - Part the vulvar labia
  - Apply sterile lubrication gel/saline onto the tip of the urinary catheter

- **Technique**

  Plastic catheter
  (under visual control)
  - Measure the required length of the urinary catheter
  - Insert the otoscope/speculum vertically into the vulva while avoiding the clitoris (lift the speculum a little)
  - Advance the otoscope/speculum horizontally until the urethral opening is reached (ventral)
  - Insert the urinary catheter under visual control
  - Advance the urinary catheter
  - Catch the urine in a sterile tube
  - Remove the urinary catheter and the otoscope/speculum

  Plastic catheter
  (under digital control)
  - Measure the required length of the urinary catheter
  - Insert the finger and urinary catheter vertically into the vulva while avoiding the clitoris
  - Advance horizontally until the urethral opening is reached
  - Insert the urinary catheter digitally into the urethra
  - Advance the urinary catheter
  - Catch the urine in a sterile tube
  - Remove the urinary catheter

Urinary Catheter in the Female Dog and Cat: Metal Catheter

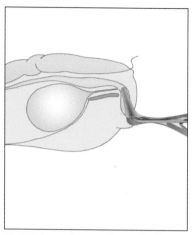

Fig 6.61 Insert the speculum vertically

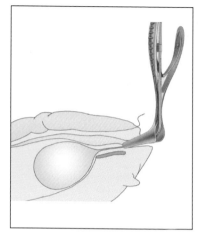

Fig 6.62 Advance the speculum horizontally

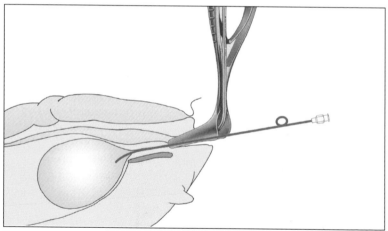

Fig 6.63 Insert the metal catheter under visual control

Method

- **Preparation**
    - Standing, sternal/prone position
    - Part the vulvar labia
    - Apply sterile lubrication gel onto the urinary catheter

- **Technique**
    - Insert the speculum vertically, then horizontally into the vulva while avoiding the clitoris
    - Spread the speculum
    - Insert the urinary catheter ventrally under visual control

Complications

- Perforation of the urethra/bladder
- Infection

Cystocentesis

Indication

- Sterile urine sampling
- Relief of pressure in case of urethral obstruction (male cat)

Cystocentesis

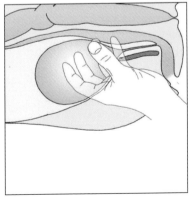

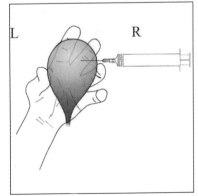

Fig 6.64 Cystocentesis while standing (lateral view)

Fig 6.65 Cystocentesis while standing (dorsal view)

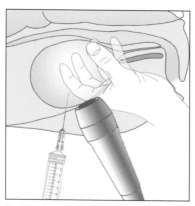

Fig 6.66 Cystocentesis under ultrasound
guidance (standing)

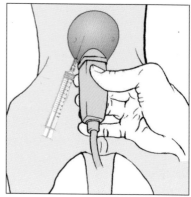

Fig 6.67 Cystocentesis under ultrasound
guidance (lying)

Method

- **Preparation**
  - Standing/dorsal position
  - Separate fur and disinfect skin

- **Technique**

  Standing
  - Fixate the urinary bladder manually
  - Insert the hypodermic needle with an attached syringe between
    your middle and ring finger through the lateral abdominal wall
    towards the thumb of the holding hand
  - Aspirate
  - Remove the syringe with the hypodermic needle while
    maintaining the insertion angle

  Dorsal position
  - Fixate the urinary bladder with the ultrasound probe
  - Puncture the urinary bladder paramedian under ultrasound
    guidance
  - Aspirate
  - Remove the syringe with the hypodermic needle while
    maintaining the insertion angle

Complications

- Perforation of the intestine
- Perforation of the aorta
- Infection

Abdominocentesis

Indication

- Abdominal effusion

Abdominocentesis

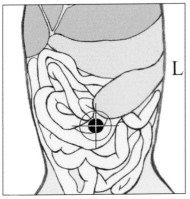

Fig 6.68 Puncture site

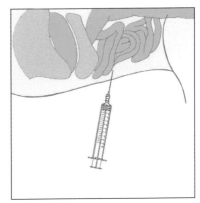

Fig 6.69 Abdominal puncture

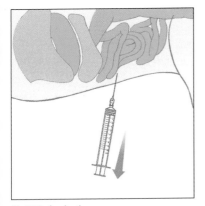

Fig 6.70 Aspiration

Method

- **Preparation**
  - Lateral recumbency
  - Clip and disinfect fur

- **Technique**
  - Possible evacuation of the urinary bladder required
  - Puncture the abdominal wall paramedian and caudal of the umbilicus (syringe with attached hypodermic needle)
  - Direct the puncture needle towards caudal
  - Aspirate
  - Remove the syringe and needle

Complications

- Splenic puncture
- Intestinal puncture
- Puncture of the urinary bladder
- Peritonitis

Further Urological Examination Methods

- **Laboratory investigations**
  - Blood
  - Urine

- **Function tests**
  - Creatinine clearance
  - Function tests for the adrenal glands
  - Water deprivation test (diabetes insipidus)

- **Laparoscopy**
  - Laparotomy

7 Gynaecological Examination Methods

Case History

Principal Symptoms

- Polydipsia
- Polyuria
- Vaginal discharge
- Behavioural changes
- Irregular oestrus cycle
- Mammary discharge

Inspection

Indication

- Part of the general examination

Inspection

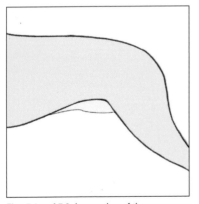

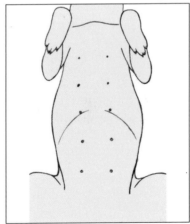

Figs 7.1 and 7.2 Inspection of the mammary strip

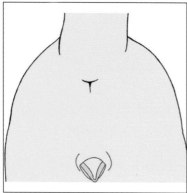

Fig 7.3 Inspection of the vulva

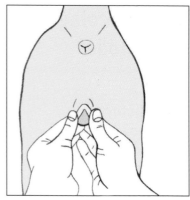

Fig 7.4 Inspection/examination of the vulva

Method

- **Technique**
    - Observe the body posture/stance, nutritional status and respiration at rest
    - Inspect the mammary glands
    - Inspect/examine the vulva

Findings

- **Physiological**
    - Costoabdominal respiration/respiration rate 10–30/min

- **Pathological**

    Mammary glands
    - Discharge/inflammation (mastitis)
    - Tumour
    - Galactorrhoea/pseudo pregnancy

    Vulva
    - Discharge (vulvitis/vaginitis, pyometra, haemometra, mucometra)
    - Tumour
    - Vaginal prolapse

Palpation

Indication

- Part of the general examination

Palpation

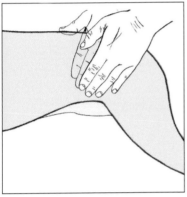

Fig 7.5 Palpation of the uterus

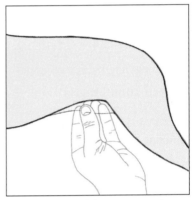

Fig 7.6 Palpation of the mammary strip

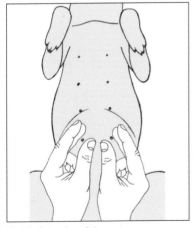

Fig 7.7 Palpation of the teats

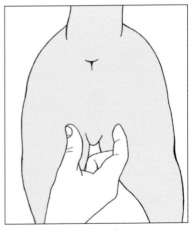

Fig 7.8 Palpation of the vulva

Method

- **Technique**

  Uterus
  - Feel the uterus (palpable during pregnancy or if there is a pathological change)

  Vulva
  - Feel the vulva externally

  Mammary strip
  - Feel along the whole length of the mammary strip and all teats including the lymph nodes

- **Evaluation criteria**
  - Size, shape, symmetry, position, consistency

Findings

- **Physiological**
  - Nothing abnormal to detect (NAD)

- **Pathological**

  Uterus
  - Pregnancy
  - Pyometra, haemometra, mucometra
  - Tumour

  Mammary glands
  - Discharge/inflammation (mastitis)
  - Tumour
  - Galactorrhoea/pseudo pregnancy

  Vulva
  - Discharge
  - Tumour
  - Vaginal prolapse

X-Ray Study

Indication

- Abdomen: suspected uterine disease or pregnancy
- Thorax: exclusion of metastasis in case of mammary masses

X-Ray Study

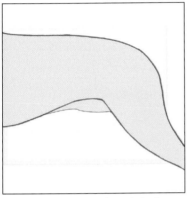

Fig 7.9 Abdomen/pelvis (lateral view)

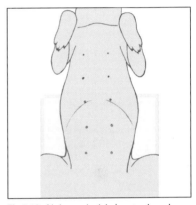

Fig 7.10 Abdomen/pelvis (ventrodorsal view)

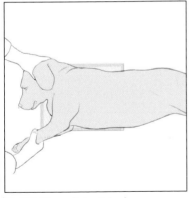

Fig 7.11 Thorax (lateral view)

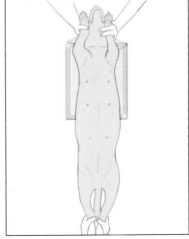

Fig 7.12 Thorax (ventrodorsal view)

Method

- **Technique**
  - Perform a risk/benefit assessment (if the patient is dyspnoeic)
  - Plan and agree the proposed procedure with colleagues and owners
  - Fully inform the owner (consider asking questions about pregnancy and age range)
  - Handle the patient calmly and in a coordinated manner
  - Consider distracting the patient
  - Take two views if at all possible

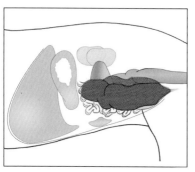

Fig 7.13 Pyometra

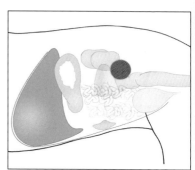

Fig 7.14 Ovarian tumour

Findings

- **Physiological**

  Uterus (non-pregnant)
  - Not visible on X-rays

  Uterus (pregnant)
  - Visible from about day 40 (skeletal ossification of the foetuses)

- **Pathological**

  Uterus
  - Uterine enlargement (endometritis, pyometra, haemometra, mucometra)
  - Tumours

  Ovaries
  - Tumours

  Thorax
  - Metastasis (mammary carcinoma)

Endoscopy: Vaginoscopy

Indication

- Position of the cervix during complications in parturition
- Suspected tumour

Vaginoscopy

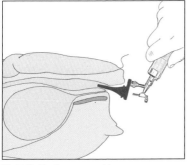

Fig 7.15 Vaginoscopy with an otoscope

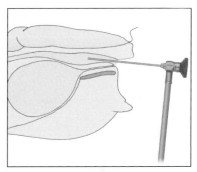

Fig 7.16 Vaginoscopy with a rigid endoscope

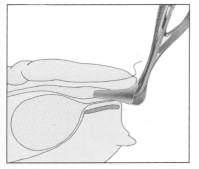

Fig 7.17 Vaginoscopy with a speculum/light source

Method

- **Preparation**
  - Standing, sternal position, parting of the vulva
  - Apply some sterile lubrication gel onto the vaginoscope

- **Technique**
  - Insert the vaginoscope vertically, then advance it horizontally into the vulva while avoiding the clitoris

Ultrasound Examination

Indication

- Pregnancy diagnosis
- Suspected uterine/ovarian disease

Ultrasound Examination: Ovaries

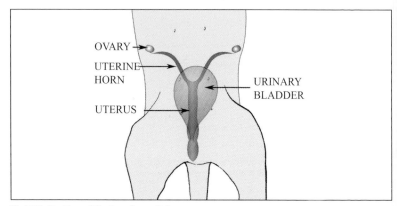

Fig 7.18 Position of the female genital organs

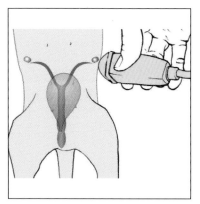

Fig 7.19 Ultrasound (longitudinal axis)

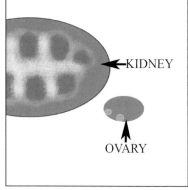

Fig 7.20 Ultrasonic pattern of the ovary

Ultrasound: Uterus

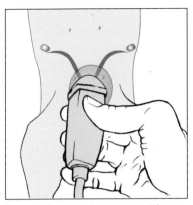

Fig 7.21 Ultrasound (transverse axis)

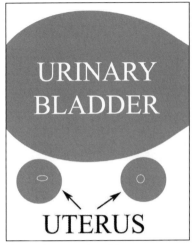

Fig 7.22 Cross section of the uterus

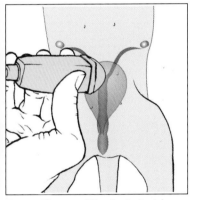

Fig 7.23 Ultrasound (longitudinal axis)

Method

- **Preparation**
    - Dorsal position
    - Clip fur as required
    - Ultrasound gel
    - Sector/linear transducer 5–7.5 MHz

- **Technique**
    - Place the probe perpendicular to the abdomen
    - Turn probe by 90°

Findings

- **Physiological**
    - Nothing abnormal to detect (NAD)
    - Pregnancy confirmation from day 25–30

- **Pathological**

    Ovaries
    - Tumour
    - Cysts

    Uterus
    - Cystic endometrial hyperplasia and endometritis
    - Pyometra/haemometra
    - Mucometra
    - Tumour
    - Rupture

Biopsy: Vaginal Smear

Indication

- Oestrus determination (dog)

Vaginal smear

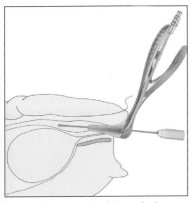

Fig 7.24 Swab sample of the vaginal
mucosa

Method

- **Preparation**
  - Standing, sternal position, parting of the vulva
  - Apply sterile lubrication gel onto the speculum

- **Technique**
  - Insert the speculum vertically, then advance it horizontally into the vulva while avoiding the clitoris
  - Take multiple smear samples of the vaginal mucosa with a swab

Further Gynaecological Examination Methods

- Laboratory examinations
- Blood
- Urine

8 Andrological Examination Methods

Case History

Principal Symptoms

- Stranguria
- Pollakisuria
- Haematuria
- Tenesmus
- Faecal impaction

- Haematochezia
- Penile discharge
- Erectile dysfunction
- Testicular enlargement/painfulness

Inspection

Indication

- Part of the general examination

Inspection

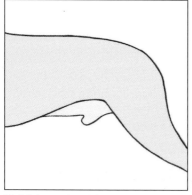

Fig 8.1 Inspection of the penis

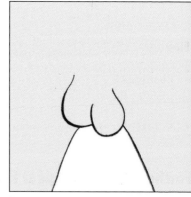

Fig 8.2 Inspection of the perineum and scrotum

Inspection

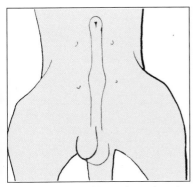

Fig 8.3 Inspection of the groin, penis and scrotum

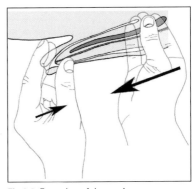

Fig 8.4 Extrusion of the penis

Method

- **Technique**
  - Observe the body posture/stance, nutritional status and respiration at rest
  - Inspect the scrotum
  - Inspect the penis
  - Inspect the groin
  - Inspect the perineum

Findings

- **Physiological**
  - Nothing abnormal to detect (NAD)

- **Pathological**

  Scrotum
  - Scrotal enlargement
  - Testicular enlargement
  - Dermatitis

  Penis
  - Discharge (urinary incontinence, balanoposthitis)
  - Tumour
  - Phimosis/paraphimosis

  Perineum/groin
  - Hernia

Palpation

Indication

• Part of the general examination

Palpation

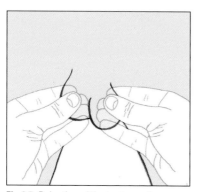

Fig 8.5 Palpation of the testes and epididymes

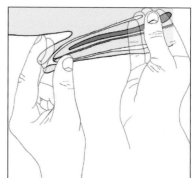

Fig 8.6 Palpation of the penis

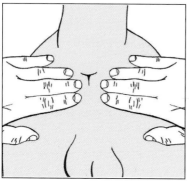

Fig 8.7 Palpation of the perineum

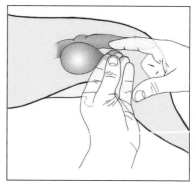

Fig 8.8 Palpation of the prostate

Method

- **Technique**

  Testes
  - Feel the testes and epididymes

  Penis
  - Feel the penile structures

  Prostate
  - Feel the prostate from rectal and abdominal

  Perineum
  - Feel the perineal muscles externally and rectally

- **Evaluation criteria**
  - Size, shape, symmetry, position, consistency

Findings

- **Physiological**
  - Nothing abnormal to detect (NAD)

- **Pathological**

  Testes
  - Inflammation (orchitis)
  - Tumour
  - Cryptorchism
  - Testicular torsion

  Penis
  - Balanoposthitis
  - Tumour

  Prostate
  - Prostatic enlargement

  Perineum
  - Perineal hernia

X-Ray Study

Indication

- Suspected prostatic enlargement

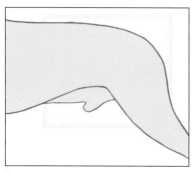

Fig 8.9 Abdomen/pelvis (lateral view)

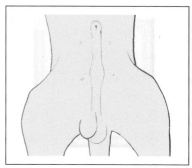

Fig 8.10 Abdomen/pelvis (dorsoventral view)

Method

- **Technique**
  - Projection of two views if at all possible

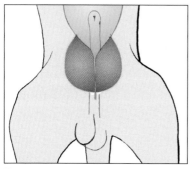

Fig 8.11 Prostatic enlargement

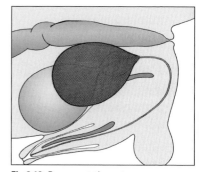

Fig 8.12 Paraprostatic cyst

Findings

- **Physiological**
  - Nothing abnormal to detect (NAD)

- **Pathological**
  Prostate
  - Prostatic enlargement
  - Paraprostatic cyst

Ultrasound Examination

Indication

- Prostatic disease
- Testicular disease and abdominal localisation of a cryptorchid testicle

Ultrasound Examination

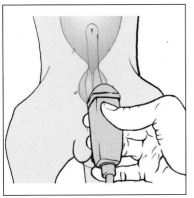

Fig 8.13 Ultrasound (longitudinal axis)

Fig 8.14 Prostate

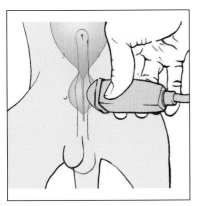

Fig 8.15 Ultrasound (transverse axis)

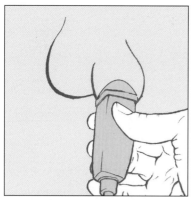

Fig 8.16 Ultrasound examination of the testes

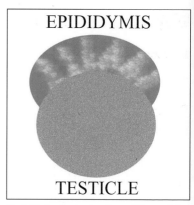

Fig 8.17 Anatomical regions of the testicle (cross section)

Method

- **Preparation**
  - Dorsal position/lateral recumbency
  - Clip fur as required
  - Ultrasound gel
  - Sector/linear transducer 5–7.5 MHz

- **Technique**
  - Place the probe perpendicular to the abdomen
  - Turn the probe by 90°

Findings

- **Physiological**
  - Nothing abnormal to detect (NAD)

- **Pathological**

  Prostate
  - Prostatic hypertrophy
  - Prostatitis
  - Prostatic cysts
  - Paraprostatic cysts
  - Prostate carcinoma

  Testicle
  - Orchitis
  - Hydrocele/spermatocele
  - Testicular torsion
  - Tumour

Biopsy: Fine Needle Aspiration Biopsy

Indication

- Suspected prostatic tumour

Biopsy of the Prostate

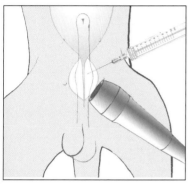 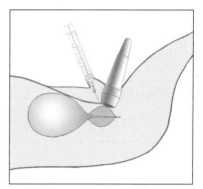

Fig 8.18 Biopsy of the prostate (ventral view)

Fig 8.19 Biopsy of the prostate (lateral view)

Method

- **Preparation**
  - Blood laboratory analysis including coagulation status
  - Dorsal position
  - Sedation/general anaesthesia
  - Clip fur/disinfect skin
  - Ultrasound examination

- **Technique**
  - Puncture the prostate percutaneously under ultrasound guidance
  - Aspirate
  - Remove the biopsy needle
  - Check the biopsy site with the ultrasound (haemorrhage)

Complications

- Haemorrhage
- Infection

9 Orthopaedic Examination Methods

Case History

Principal Symptoms

- Lameness

Inspection

Indication

- Part of the general examination

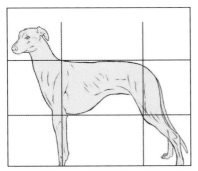

Fig 9.1 Body and limb posture/position (lateral)

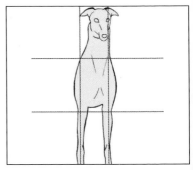

Fig 9.2 Body and limb posture/position (anterior)

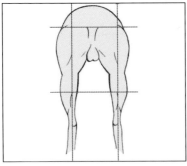

Fig 9.3 Body and limb posture/position (posterior)

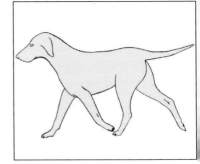

Fig 9.4 Gait analysis

Method

- **Technique**
  - Observe the body posture
  - Observe the limb posture/position
  - Observe the body condition/constitution
  - Observe the movement pattern (walking, trotting, running)

Findings

- **Physiological**
  - Nothing abnormal to detect (NAD)

- **Pathological**

  Body posture/position
  - Lowering of the head (cervical spine)
  - Lateral recumbency
  - Sternal/prone position
  - Sitting (painfulness in the pelvis or hind limbs)
  - Dorsal position (painfulness in the abdomen)
  - Praying position (painfulness in the cranial abdomen)

  Limb posture/position
  - Uneven weight distribution (painfulness)
  - Malposition
    - Valgus/varus position
    - Abduction/adduction
    - Hyperextension/hyperflexion
    - Torsion/rotation
    - Supination/pronation

  Muscle tone
  - Atrophy
  - Contracture

  Gait
  - Supportive limb lameness (Grade I–IV)
  - Hanging limb lameness (Grade I–IV)
  - Head nodding (towards healthy side)
  - Hip swing (hip joint disease)
  - Locking of the knee joint (patella luxation)
  - Inner/outer rotation (elbow, knee, hip joint disease)
  - Walking diagonally
  - Elevation/lowering of the head (spinal disease)
  - Dragging of the paw (neurological disease)

Palpation: Skull

Indication

- Part of the general orthopaedic examination

Palpation: Skull

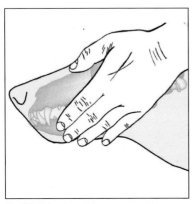

Fig 9.5 Palpation of the upper and lower jaw

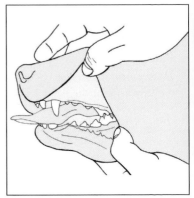

Fig 9.6 Palpation and inspection of the teeth

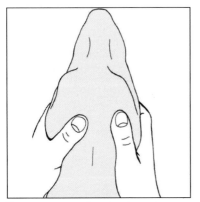

Fig 9.7 Palpation of the head muscles

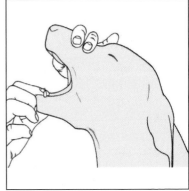

Fig 9.8 Opening of the lower jaw

Palpation: Spine

Indication

- Part of the general orthopaedic examination
- Suspected spinal disease

Palpation: Spine

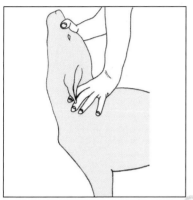

Fig 9.9 Extension of the cervical spine

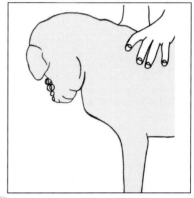

Fig 9.10 Flexion of the cervical spine

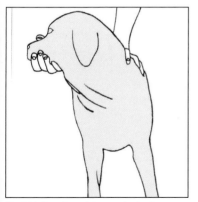

Fig 9.11 Rotation of the cervical spine

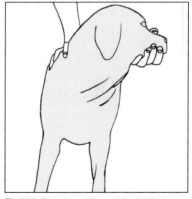

Fig 9.12 Rotation of the cervical spine

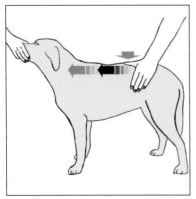

Fig 9.13 Palpation of the spine from caudal

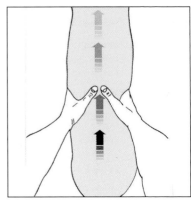

Fig 9.14 Palpation of the spine from caudal

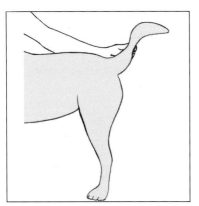

Fig 9.15 Lifting of the tail

Palpation: Forelimb

Indication

- Lameness of the forelimb
- Part of the general orthopaedic examination

Palpation: Forelimb

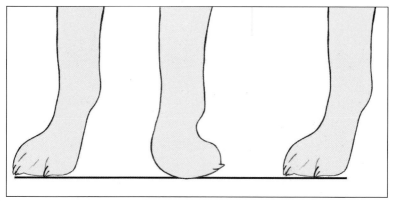

Fig 9.16 Correction reaction in the forelimb after the paws are turned into the knuckling position

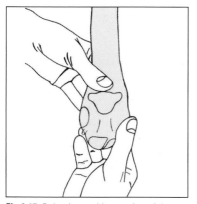

Fig 9.17 Palpation and inspection of the pads

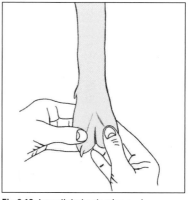

Fig 9.18 Interdigital palpation and inspection

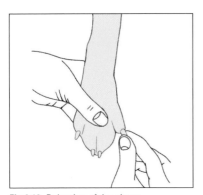

Fig 9.19 Palpation of the claws

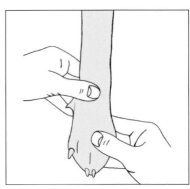

Fig 9.20 Palpation of the metacarpals

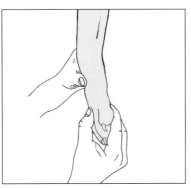

Fig 9.21 Palpation of the metacarpals

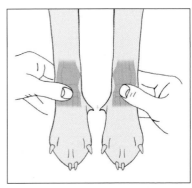

Fig 9.22 Comparative palpation of the carpal joint

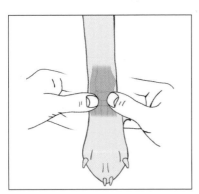

Fig 9.23 Detailed palpation of the carpal joint

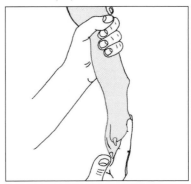

Fig 9.24 Extension of the carpal joint

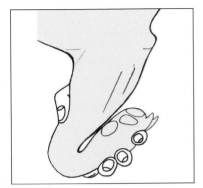

Fig 9.25 Flexion of the carpal joint

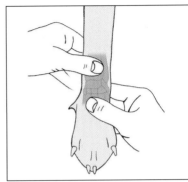

Fig 9.26 Palpation of the stability of the carpal bones

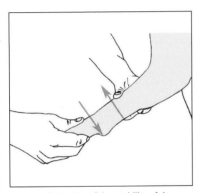

Fig 9.27 Palpation of the stability of the carpal bones

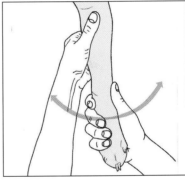

Fig 9.28 Palpation of the lateral stability of the carpal joint

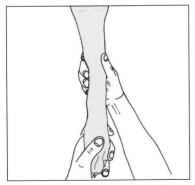

Fig 9.29 Palpation of the radius and ulna

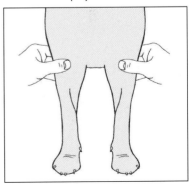

Fig 9.30 Comparative palpation of the elbow joint

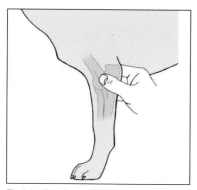

Fig 9.31 Detailed palpation of the elbow joint

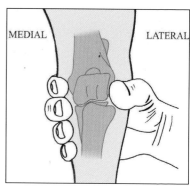

Fig 9.32 Pressure palpation of the medial anatomical landmarks

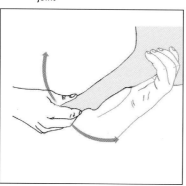

Fig 9.33 Extension and flexion of the elbow joint

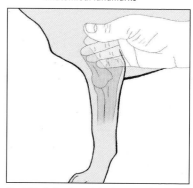

Fig 9.34 Palpation of the humerus (from medial)

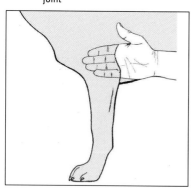

Fig 9.35 Palpation of the brachial plexus

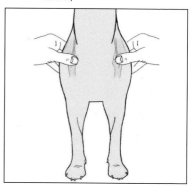

Fig 9.36 Comparative palpation of the shoulder joint

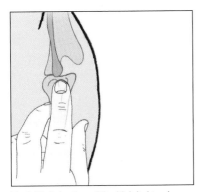

Fig 9.37 Palpation of the bicipital tendon

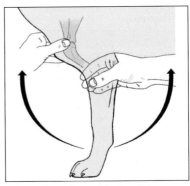

Fig 9.38 Extension and flexion of the shoulder joint

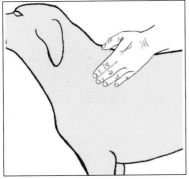

Fig 9.39 Comparative palpation of the scapula

Palpation: Hind Limb

Indication

- Hind limb lameness
- Part of the general orthopaedic examination

Palpation: Hind Limb

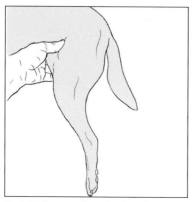

Fig 9.40 Comparative palpation of the femoral pulse

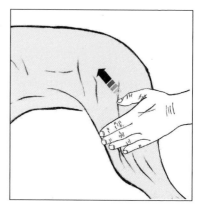

Fig 9.41 Palpation of the muscle tone

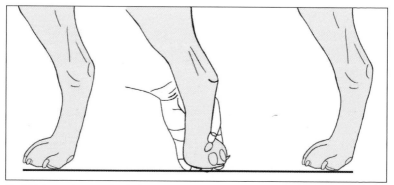

Fig 9.42 Correction reaction in the hind limb after the paws are turned into the knuckling position

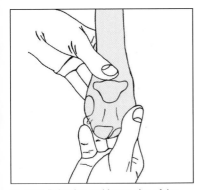

Fig 9.43 Palpation and inspection of the pads

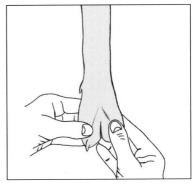

Fig 9.44 Interdigital palpation and inspection

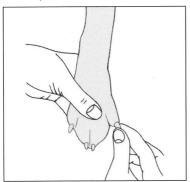

Fig 9.45 Palpation of the claws

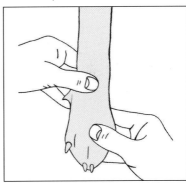

Fig 9.46 Palpation of the metatarsals

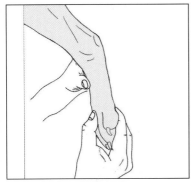

Fig 9.47 Palpation of the metatarsals

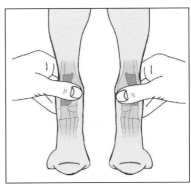

Fig 9.48 Comparative palpation of the tarsal joint

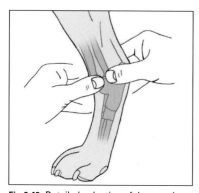

Fig 9.49 Detailed palpation of the tarsal joint

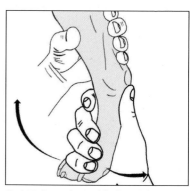

Fig 9.50 Extension and flexion of the tarsal joint

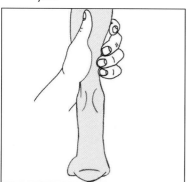

Fig 9.51 Palpation of the tibia

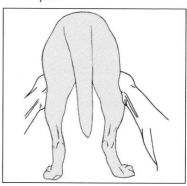

Fig 9.52 Comparative palpation of the knee joint

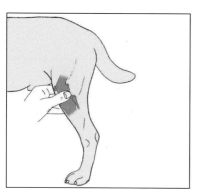

Fig 9.53 Detailed palpation of the knee joint

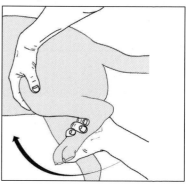

Fig 9.54 Extension and flexion of the knee joint

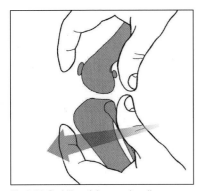

Fig 9.55 Stability of the cruciate ligament: drawer test

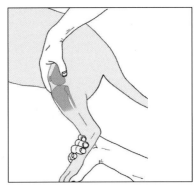

Fig 9.56 Stability of the cruciate ligament: tibial compression test (1)

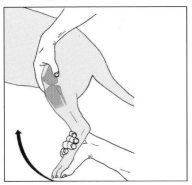

Fig 9.57 Stability of the cruciated ligament: tibial compression test (2)

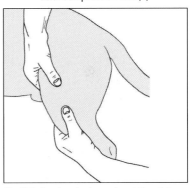

Fig 9.58 Testing the lateral stability of the knee joint

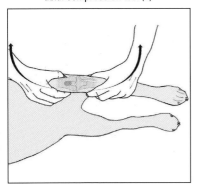

Fig 9.59 Testing the lateral stability of the knee joint

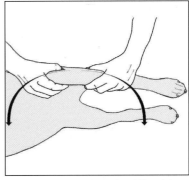

Fig 9.60 Testing the lateral stability of the knee joint

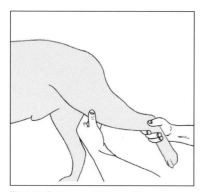

Fig 9.61 Palpation of the patella

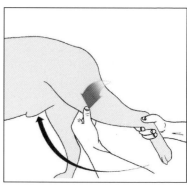

Fig 9.62 Patella: inner rotation and flexion of the limb

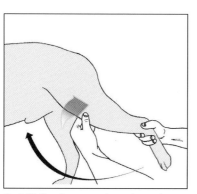

Fig 9.63 Patella: external rotation and flexion of the limb

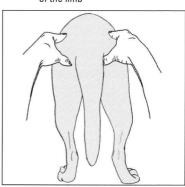

Fig 9.64 Comparative palpation of the hip

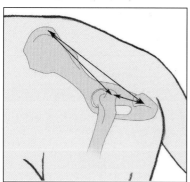

Fig 9.65 Iliac crest, ischial tuberosity, large trochanter

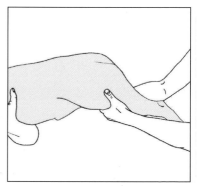

Fig 9.66 Extension of both hip joints (length comparison)

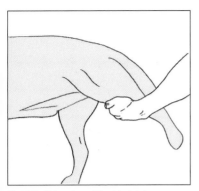

Fig 9.67 Extension of the hip joint

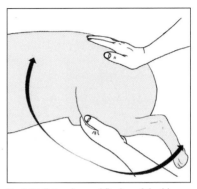

Fig 9.68 Extension and flexion of the hip joint (lateral recumbency)

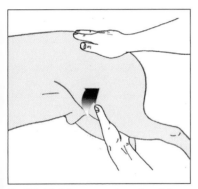

Fig 9.69 Hip joint: external rotation of the femur

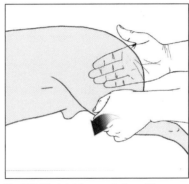

Fig 9.70 Hip joint: inner rotation of the femur

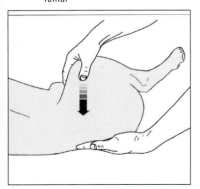

Fig 9.71 Hip joint: subluxation attempt (Ortolani manoeuvre)

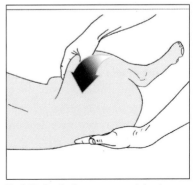

Fig 9.72 Ortolani manoeuvre: abduction, then clicking when repositioned

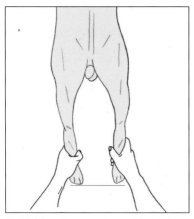

Fig 9.73 Length comparison of the hind limb

Method

- **Preparation**
  - Examine the patient while standing on the examination table, afterwards do so in lateral recumbency
  - Dorsal position for measuring the length of the hind limb
- **Evaluation criteria**
  - Size, shape, symmetry, consistency, temperature, stability, painfulness, crepitus
- **Technique**

  Skull
  - Palpate the head muscles
  - Open and close the lower jaw (jaw occlusion)

  Cervical spine
  - Extend/flex and rotate the head to both sides

  Thoracic/lumbar spine
  - Perform a pressure palpation of each vertebra from caudal to cranial

  Paw (fore and hind limbs)
  - Place them into knuckling position, evaluate the correction reaction

- Palpate/inspect the pads
- Palpate the flexor tendons
- Palpate/inspect interdigitally
- Palpate the claws/toes, extend/flex the toes
- Palpate the sesamoids
- Palpate the metacarpals/metatarsals

Carpal joint
- Perform a comparative palpation (joint effusion)
- Perform a detailed palpation
- Extend/flex
- Check the stability (attempt to open the joint into all directions)

Radius/ulna
- Perform a pressure palpation (periosteal stimulus)

Elbow joint
- Perform a comparative palpation (joint effusion)
- Perform a detailed palpation (lateral epicondyle, medial epicondyle and olecranal tuber in one line)
- Extend/flex, perform inward and outward rotation
- Anconeal process: perform a pressure palpation
- Medial coronoid process: perform a pressure palpation distal of the medial epicondyle while flexing and rotating the lower limb inwards

Humerus
- Perform a pressure palpation (periosteal stimulus)

Shoulder joint
- Perform a comparative palpation (joint effusion)
- Perform a detailed palpation (acromion, greater tuberosity)
- Extend/flex, perform inward and outward rotation
- Bicipital tendon: perform comparative hyperflexion of the shoulder joint, perform a pressure palpation of the bicipital tendon

Scapula
- Perform a comparative palpation

Axilla
- Perform a comparative palpation of the brachial plexus

Tarsal joint
- Perform a comparative palpation (joint effusion)
- Perform a detailed palpation

- Extend/flex
- Check the lateral stability: abduct and adduct

Tibia/fibula
- Perform a pressure palpation (medial)
- Perform a pressure palpation of the lateral malleolus

Knee joint
- Perform a comparative palpation (joint effusion)
- Perform a detailed palpation (tibial tuberosity, patella, medial and lateral tibial and femoral condyles)
- Extend/flex
- Check the stability of the cruciate ligament:
  1. Drawer test: shift the tibia towards cranial (anatomical landmarks: tibial tuberosity and tibial condyle) while fixating the femur (anatomical landmarks: patella and femoral condyle) and flexing the joint moderately
  2. Tibial compression test: rest the forefinger of one hand over the patella on the tibial tuberosity and check for any tibial forward motion while flexing the tarsal joint
- Check the stability of the collateral ligaments: abduct/adduct

Patella
- Perform a comparative palpation
- Apply lateral and medial patellar pressure during the inner and external rotation, extension and flexion of the joint

Femur
- Perform a pressure palpation (periosteal stimulus)

Hip joint
- Perform a comparative palpation of the distances between the bony anatomical landmarks (iliac crest, ischial tuberosity, large trochanter)
- Hyperextend both hip joints while the patient is standing
- Extend, flex and rotate the hip inwards and outwards while the patient is in lateral recumbency
- Subluxation attempt (Ortolani test): apply some pressure onto the femur/hip joint in the longitudinal axis (dorsal position with a 90° flexed knee joint). Abduct the limb (clicking sound during reposition)

Inner thigh
- Palpate the pulse: femoral artery
- Palpate the pectineal muscle

Findings

- **Physiological**
  - Nothing abnormal to detect (NAD)
- **Pathological**

  Skull
  - Atrophy of the head muscles
  - Luxation/fracture of the lower jaw
  - Lockjaw
  - Osteodystrophia fibrosa/rubber jaw
  - Tumour

  Spine
  - Vertebral lesion, spinal lesion, meningitis, meningoencephalitis

  Paw
  - Scuffed and torn claws
  - Fracture, luxation
  - Inflammation, tumour, foreign body

  Carpal joint
  - Arthritis, arthrosis
  - Fracture, luxation
  - Ligament rupture (hyperflexion), tendon rupture
  - Tumour

  Radius/ulna
  - Fracture, luxation
  - Panosteitis
  - Radius curvus
  - Muscular atrophy
  - Tumour

  Elbow joint
  - Fracture, luxation
  - Arthritis, arthrosis
  - Tumour
    - Isolated, fragmented medial coronoid process
    - Isolated anconeal process

  Humerus
  - Fracture, luxation
  - Panosteitis
  - Muscular atrophy
  - Tumour

Shoulder joint
- Fracture, luxation
- Arthritis, arthrosis
- Tumour
- Muscular atrophy
- Bicipial tendon rupture, tendovaginitis

Scapula
- Fracture, luxation
- Muscle contracture: supra-/infraspinous muscle
- Muscular atrophy

Axilla
- Brachial plexus: tumour, severance
- Lymphadenopathy

Tarsal joint
- Fracture, luxation
- Arthritis, arthrosis
- Ligament or tendon rupture
- Tumour
- Muscular atrophy
- Hyperextension syndrome

Tibia/fibula
- Fracture, luxation
- Panosteitis
- Tumour

Knee joint
- Fracture, luxation
- Arthritis, arthrosis
- Ligament rupture (cruciate ligaments, collateral ligaments)
- Tumour
- Patellar luxation or fracture
- Patellar tendon rupture

Femur
- Fracture
- Muscle contracture: gracilis muscle, quadriceps muscle
- Muscle atrophy
- Tumour

Hip joint
- Fracture, luxation
- Arthritis, arthrosis
- Pectineal muscle: tension

X-Ray Study: Skull

Indication

- Dysphagia

X-Ray Study: Head

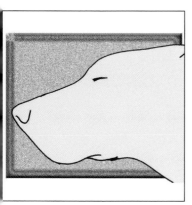

Fig 9.74 Head (lateral view)

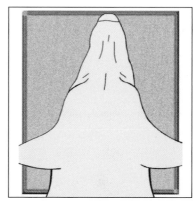

Fig 9.75 Head (dorsoventral view)

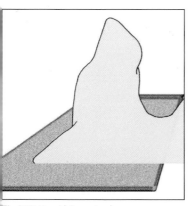

Fig 9.76 Head (sinus view)

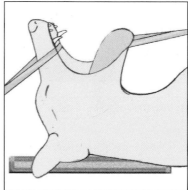

Fig 9.77 Head (rostrocaudal/bullar view)

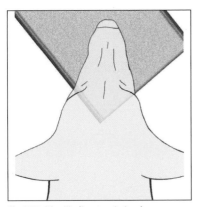

Fig 9.78 Maxilla (intraoral plate)

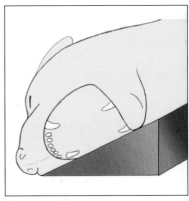

Fig 9.79 Maxilla (oblique view)

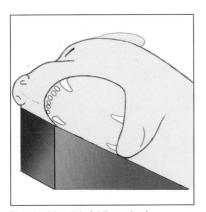

Fig 9.80 Mandible (oblique view)

X- Ray Study: Spine

Indication

- Spinal disease

X-Ray Study: Spine

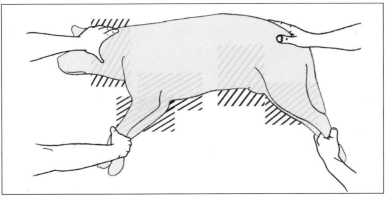

Fig 9.81 Padding

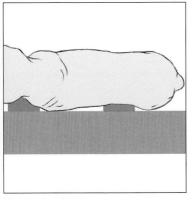

Fig 9.82 Padding

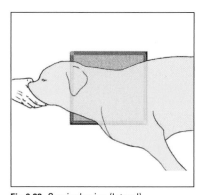

Fig 9.83 Cervical spine (lateral)

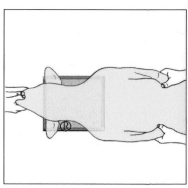

Fig 9.84 Cervical spine (ventrodorsal)

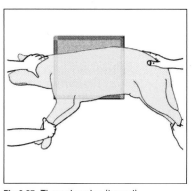

Fig 9.85 Thoracic spine (lateral)

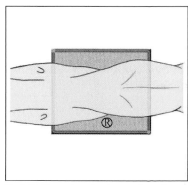

Fig 9.86 Thoracic spine (ventrodorsal)

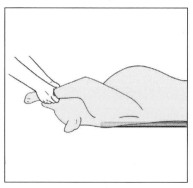

Fig 9.87 Thoracic spine (ventrodorsal),
view from lateral

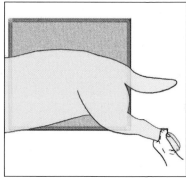

Fig 9.88 Lumbar spine (lateral)

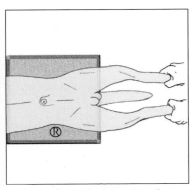

Fig 9.89 Lumbar spine (ventrodorsal)

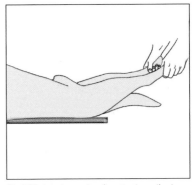

Fig 9.90 Lumbar spine (ventrodorsal), view from lateral

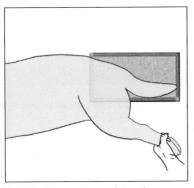

Fig 9.91 Coccygeal spine (lateral)

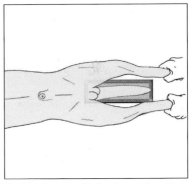

Fig 9.92 Coccygeal spine (ventrodorsal)

X- Ray Study: Forelimb

Indication

- Lameness of unknown origin
- Elbow dysplasia (early diagnosis)

X-Ray Study: Forelimb

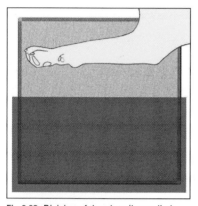

Fig 9.93 Division of the plate (lower limb lateral)

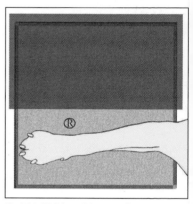

Fig 9.94 Division of the plate (lower limb dorsoventral)

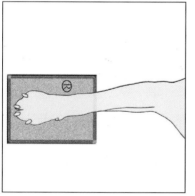

Fig 9.95 Paw (dorsoventral/craniocaudal)

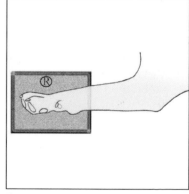

Fig 9.96 Paw (lateral)

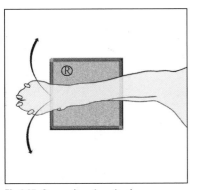

Fig 9.97 Carpus (tension view)

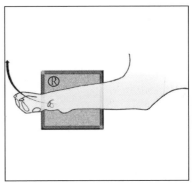

Fig 9.98 Carpus (tension view)

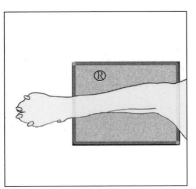

Fig 9.99 Radius/ulna (dorsoventral)

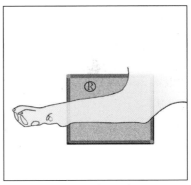

Fig 9.100 Radius/ulna (lateral)

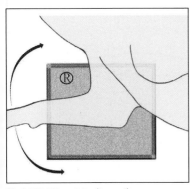

Fig 9.101 Elbow joint (lateral)

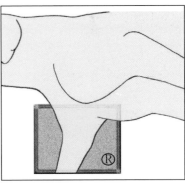

Fig 9.102 Elbow joint (lateral)

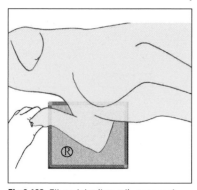

Fig 9.103 Elbow joint (lateral), anconeal process

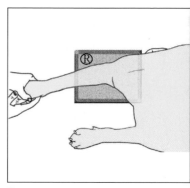

Fig 9.104 Elbow joint (dorsoventral)

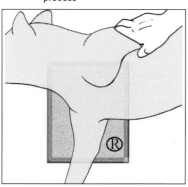

Fig 9.105 Humerus (lateral)

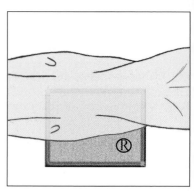

Fig 9.106 Humerus (ventrodorsal)

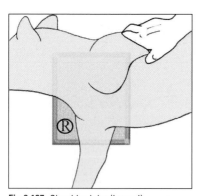

Fig 9.107 Shoulder joint (lateral)

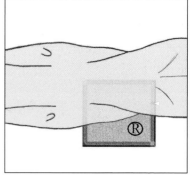

Fig 9.108 Shoulder joint (ventrodorsal)

X- Ray Study: Hind Limb

Indication

- Lameness of unknown origin
- Hip dysplasia (HD) (early diagnosis)

X-Ray Study: Hind Limb

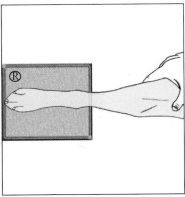

Fig 9.109 Paw (dorsoventral/craniocaudal)

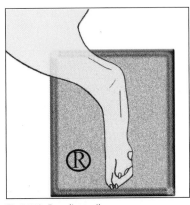

Fig 9.110 Paw (lateral)

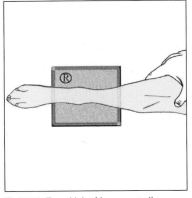

Fig 9.111 Tarsal joint (dorsoventral)

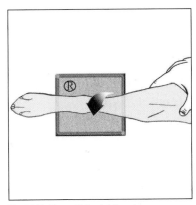

Fig 9.112 Tarsal joint (oblique): osteochondrosis dissecans (OCD)

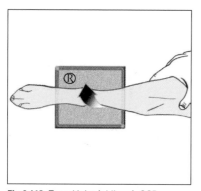

Fig 9.113 Tarsal joint (oblique): OCD

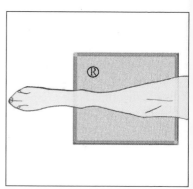

Fig 9.114 Tibia/fibula (dorsoventral)

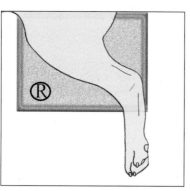

Fig 9.115 Tibia/fibula (lateral)

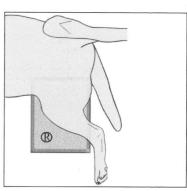

Fig 9.116 Knee joint (lateral)

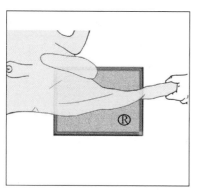

Fig 9.117 Knee joint (dorsoventral)

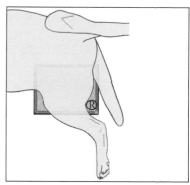

Fig 9.118 Femur (lateral)

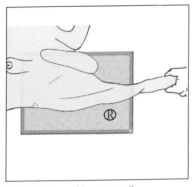

Fig 9.119 Femur (dorsoventral)

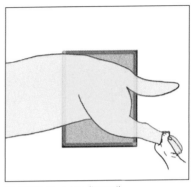

Fig 9.120 Hip joints (lateral)

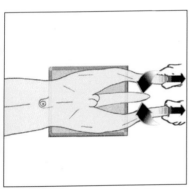

Fig 9.121 Hip joints: hip dysplasia X-rays

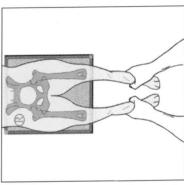

Fig 9.122 Correct position for hip dysplasia X-rays

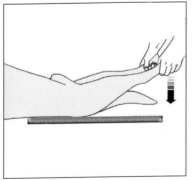

Fig 9.123 Hip joints: hip dysplasia X-rays

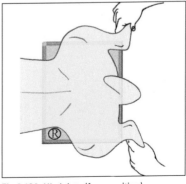

Fig 9.124 Hip joints (frog position)

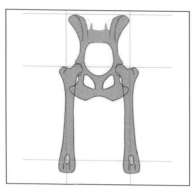

Fig 9.125 Correct position for hip dysplasia X-rays

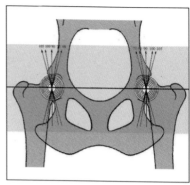

Fig 9.126 Norberg angle measurement

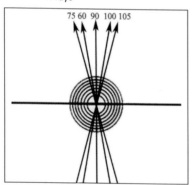

Fig 9.127 Norberg angle template

Method

- **Technique**

  General
  - Perform a risk/benefit assessment (if the patient is dyspnoeic)
  - Plan and agree the proposed procedure with colleagues and owners
  - Fully inform the owner (consider questions regarding a possible pregnancy and age range)
  - Handle the patient calmly and in a coordinated manner
  - Consider distracting the patient
  - Take two views if at all possible (dividing the plate is possible and sensible)
  - Tension view under general anaesthetic
  - Padding

  Hip dysplasia (HD) X-rays (refer to the official KC/BVA hip dysplasia scheme)
  - Relevant documents from the Kennel Club/BVA
  - Pedigree
  - KC number
  - Tattoo number
  - Age (1–1.5 years)
  - X-ray marker with required details (including microchip)
  - Left/right marker
  - Sedation
  - Positioning:
    - Position 1: symmetrical dorsal, parallel to the table extended and inwards rotated hind limbs
    - Position 2: dorsal with symmetrically flexed (45°) hind limbs (frog position)

  Norberg angle measurement
  - Place the Norberg template onto the X-ray (onto the centre of the femoral head)
  - Measure the angle to the craniodorsal rim of the acetabulum

- **HD evaluation**

  ### No signs of HD (HD 0 A1/A2)
  - Joint space: narrow, congruent
  - Norberg angle: >105°
  - Outline of the cranial aspect of the acetabulum: like a fine line
  - Acetabular rim: sharp and slightly rounded
  - Femoral head: spherical, separated from the neck, centre medial of the dorsal acetabular rim

  ### Transitional case (HD I B1/B2)
  - Joint space: diverging/incongruent TBC with Norberg angle > 105°, or Norberg angle 100–105° with minimal incongruence of the joint space

  ### Mild HD (HD II C1/C2)
  - Joint space: incongruent
  - Norberg angle: >100°
  - Craniodorsal rim of the acetabulum: medial to the centre of the femoral head
  - Craniodorsal rim of acetabulum: flattened

  ### Moderate HD (HD III D1/D2)
  - Joint space: clearly incongruent
  - Norberg angle: >90°
  - Craniodorsal rim of the acetabulum: medial to the centre of the femoral head
  - Craniodrosal rim of the acetabulum: flattened
  - Degenerative joint disease

  ### Severe HD (HD IV E1/E2)
  - Joint space: clearly incongruent
  - Norberg angle: <90°
  - Craniodorsal rim of the acetabulum: medial to the centre of the femoral head
  - Craniodrosal rim of the acetabulum: flattened
  - Degenerative joint disease
  - Femoral head: deformed

X-Ray Findings: Head

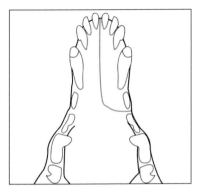

Fig 9.128 Maxillar fracture

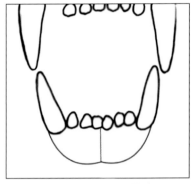

Fig 9.129 Fracture of the mandibular symphysis

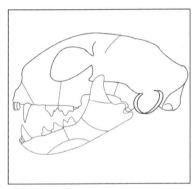

Fig 9.130 Skull fractures

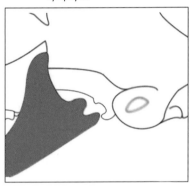

Fig 9.131 Mandibular luxation

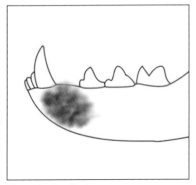

Fig 9.132 Mandibular tumour

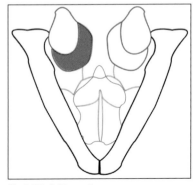

Fig 9.133 Otitis media

X-Ray Findings: Spine

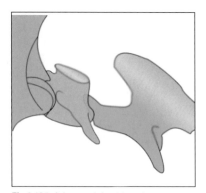

Fig 9.134 Atlantoaxial subluxation

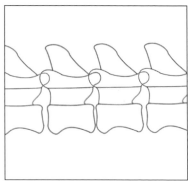

Fig 9.135 Intervertebral disc prolapse

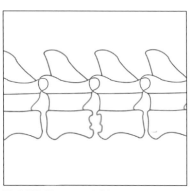

Fig 9.136 Discospondylitis

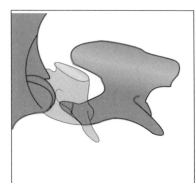

Fig 9.137 Dens axis fracture

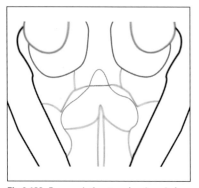

Fig 9.138 Dens axis fracture (oral cavity)

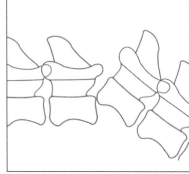

Fig 9.139 Spinal luxation fracture

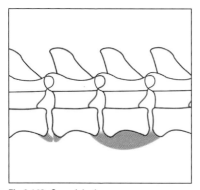

Fig 9.140 Spondylosis

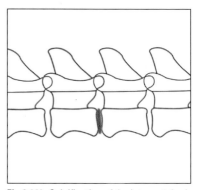

Fig 9.141 Calcification of the intervertebral disc

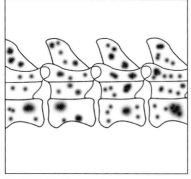

Fig 9.142 Multiple myeloma

X-Ray Findings: Paw

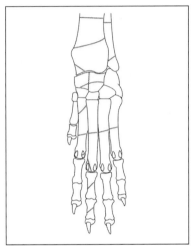

Fig 9.143 Fractures of the paw

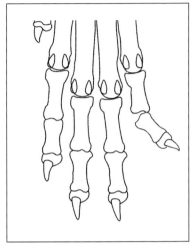

Fig 9.144 Digital luxation

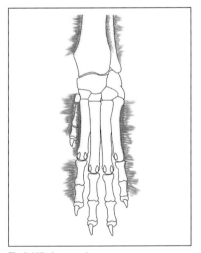

Fig 9.145 Acropachy

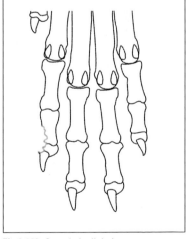

Fig 9.146 Osteolytic digital tumour

X-Ray Findings: Carpal joint

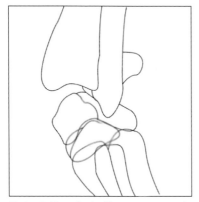

Fig 9.147 Hyperflexion/ligament rupture of the carpal joint

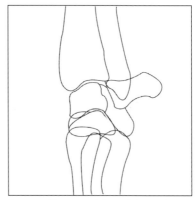

Fig 9.148 Fracture of the radial carpal bone

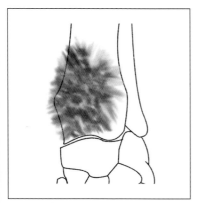

Fig 9.149 Osteosarcoma of the distal radius

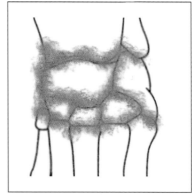

Fig 9.150 Carpal joint arthrosis

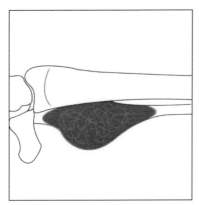

Fig 9.151 Bone cyst of the distal ulna

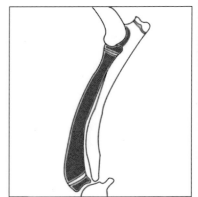

Fig 9.152 Radius curvus

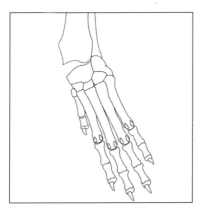

Fig 9.153 Rupture of the lateral ligament in the carpal joint

X-Ray Findings: Elbow Joint

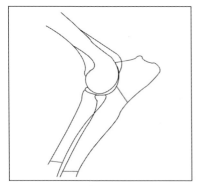

Fig 9.154 Fracture (radius/ulna)

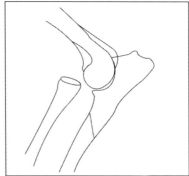

Fig 9.155 Monteggia fracture

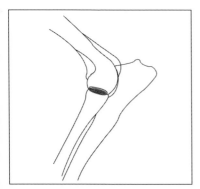

Fig 9.156 Elbow luxation

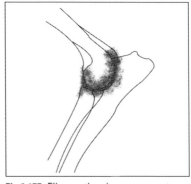

Fig 9.157 Elbow arthrosis

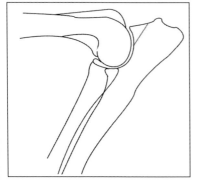

Fig 9.158 Ununited anconeal process

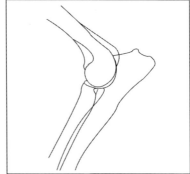

Fig 9.159 Ununited coronoid process

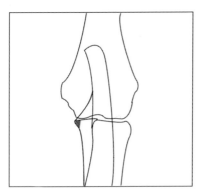

Fig 9.160 Ununited medial coronoid process

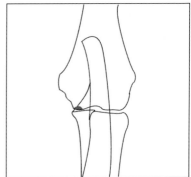

Fig 9.161 Osteochondrosis dissecans (OCD) elbow joint

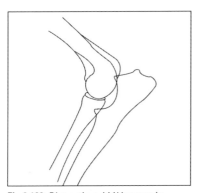

Fig 9.162 Distractio cubiti/dysostosis enchondralis

X-Ray Findings: Shoulder Joint

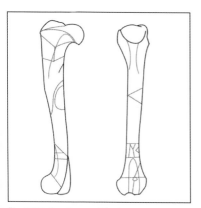

Fig 9.163 Fractures of the humerus

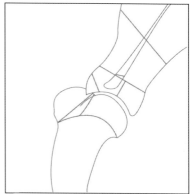

Fig 9.164 Fractures of the shoulder joint

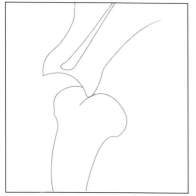

Fig 9.165a–b Luxation of the shoulder joint

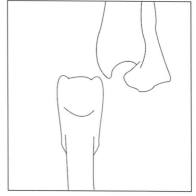

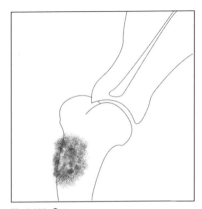

Fig 9.166 Osteosarcoma

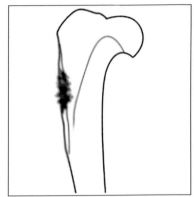

Fig 9.167 Osteomyelitis near the shoulder joint

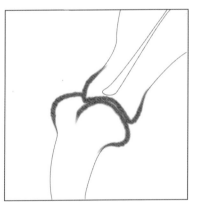

Fig 9.168 Shoulder joint arthrosis

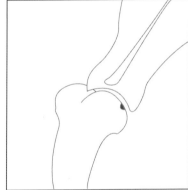

Fig 9.169 OCD Shoulder joint

X-Ray Findings: Tarsal Joint

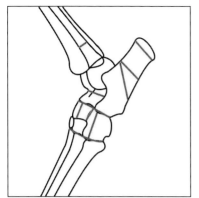

Fig 9.170 Fractures of the tarsal joint (lateral)

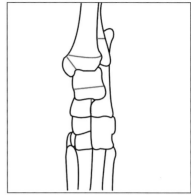

Fig 9.171 Fractures of the tarsal joint (anteroposterior)

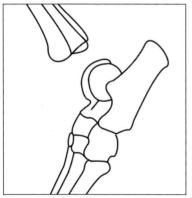

Fig 9.172 Luxation of the tibiotarsal joint

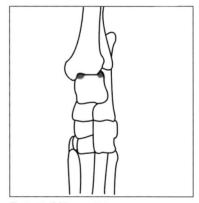

Fig 9.173 OCD tarsal joint

X-Ray Findings: Knee Joint

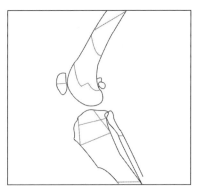

Fig 9.174 Knee joint fractures (lateral)

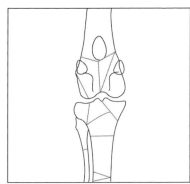

Fig 9.175 Knee joint fractures (anteroposterior)

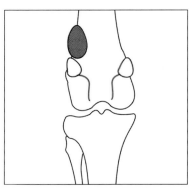

Fig 9.176 Patellar luxation towards lateral

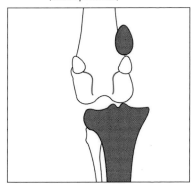

Fig 9.177 Patellar luxation towards medial

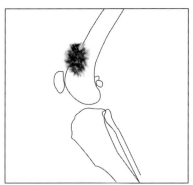

Fig 9.178 Osteosarcoma of the distal femur

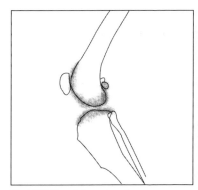

Fig 9.179 Knee joint arthrosis

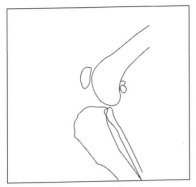

Fig 9.180 Cranial cruciate ligament rupture

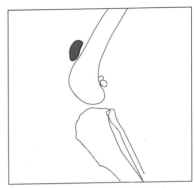

Fig 9.181 Rupture of the patellar tendon

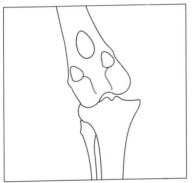

Fig 9.182 Rupture of the medial collateral ligament of the knee joint

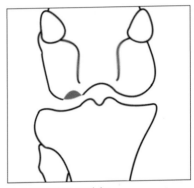

Fig 9.183 OCD knee joint

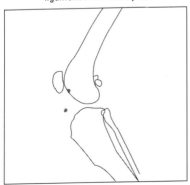

Fig 9.184 Avulsion of the long digital extensor tendon

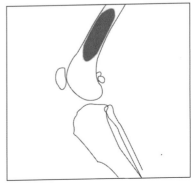

Fig 9.185 Panosteitis

X-Ray Findings: Hip Joint

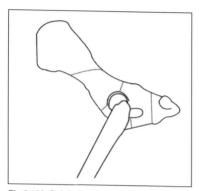

Fig 9.186 Pelvic fractures (lateral)

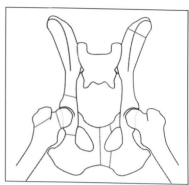

Fig 9.187 Pelvic fractures (ventrodorsal)

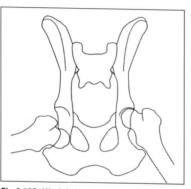

Fig 9.188 Hip joint luxation towards caudal

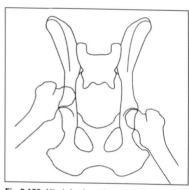

Fig 9.189 Hip joint luxation towards cranial

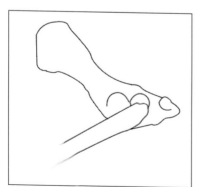

Fig 9.190 Hip joint luxation towards caudodorsal

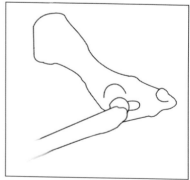

Fig 9.191 Hip joint luxation towards caudoventral

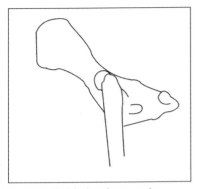

Fig 9.192 Hip joint luxation towards craniodorsal

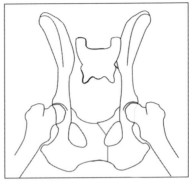

Fig 9.193 Luxation of the ileosacral joint

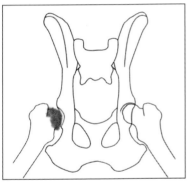

Fig 9.194 Coxarthrosis

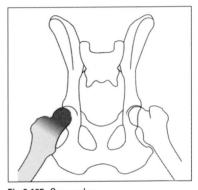

Fig 9.195 Coxa valga

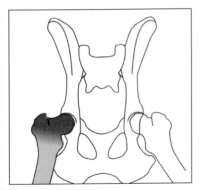

Fig 9.196 Coxa vara

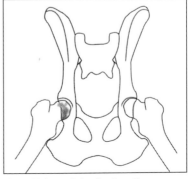

Fig 9.197 Legg-Calve-Perthes disease

Findings

- **Physiological**
  - Nothing abnormal to detect (NAD)

- **Pathological**

  Head
  - Fracture (maxillar, symphysial, skull)
  - Mandibular luxation
  - Craniomandibular osteopathy (CMO)
  - Tumour/mandibular tumour
  - Osteomyelitis
  - Sinusitis
  - Otitis media
  - Radiopaque foreign body

  Cervical spine
  - Vertebral fracture
  - Dens axis fracture
  - Luxation
  - Luxation fracture
  - Atlantoaxial subluxation
  - Wobbler syndrome
  - Vertebral disc prolapse
  - Discospondylitis/osteomyelitis
  - Deforming spondylosis
  - Spondylosis
  - Calcification of a vertebral disc
  - Tumour/multiple myeloma

  Thoracic/lumbar spine
  - Vertebral fracture
  - Luxation
  - Luxation fracture
  - Vertebral disc prolapse
  - Discospondylitis/osteomyelitis
  - Deforming spondylosis
  - Spondylosis
  - Calcification of a vertebral disc
  - Tumour/multiple myeloma
  - Lumbosacral stenosis (cauda equina syndrome)
  - Osteoporosis/-petrosis/hypervitaminosis A
  - Vertebral deformations

Paw
- Fracture/sesamoid fracture
- Luxation/digital luxation
- Tumour/osteolytic digital tumour
- Osteomyelitis
- Arthrosis
- Acropachy

Carpal joint
- Ligament rupture (hyperflexion, rupture of the lateral ligament)
- Fracture/fracture of the radial carpal bone
- Luxation
- Tumour/osteosarcoma
- Osteomyelitis
- Arthritis/arthrosis (carpal joint arthrosis)
- Bone cyst of the distal ulna
- Radius curvus

Radius/ulna
- Fracture
- Luxation (distractio cubiti/dysostosis enchondralis)
- Radius curvus/short radius syndrome/short ulna syndrome
- Tumour
- Osteomyelitis
- Panosteitis
- Metabolic disturbances (e.g., hypertrophic osteodystrophy)

Elbow joint
- Fracture (radius/ulna)
- Monteggia fracture
- Luxation
- Tumour
- Osteomyelitis
- Arthritis/arthrosis
- Elbow dysplasis (ED)
- Ununited anconeal process (UAP)
- Ununited/fragmented medial coronoid process (FCP)
- Ununited coronoid process (UCP)
- Osteochondrosis dissecans (OCD)
- Distractio cubiti/dysostosis enchondralis

Humerus
- Fracture
- Tumour
- Panosteitis
- Osteomyelitis
- Metabolic disturbances

Shoulder joint
- Fracture
- Luxation
- Tumour (osteosarcoma)
- Osteomyelitis
- Arthritis/arthrosis
- Osteochondrosis dissecans (OCD)
- Rupture of the bicipital tendon

Scapula
- Fracture
- Luxation
- Tumour

Tarsal joint
- Fracture
- Luxation
- Tumour
- Osteomyelitis
- Arthritis/arthrosis
- Osteochondrosis dissecans (OCD)
- Rupture of the Achilles tendon

Tibia/fibula
- Fracture
- Luxation
- Tumour
- Osteomyelitis
- Panosteitis
- Apophyseal fracture
- Metabolic disturbances

Knee joint
- Fracture
- Patellar luxation (towards lateral/medial)
- Tumour (osteosarcoma of the distal femur)

- Osteomyelitis
- Arthritis/arthrosis
- Cruciate ligament rupture/collateral ligament rupture (lateral/medial)/rupture of the patellar tendon
- Osteochondrosis dissecans (OCD)
- Avulsion of the long digital extensor tendon
- Panosteitis

Femur
- Fracture
- Luxation
- Tumour
- Panosteitis
- Apophyseal fracture
- Osteomyelitis
- Metabolic disturbances

Hip joint
- Fracture
- Luxation (towards caudal/cranial/caudodorsal/caudoventral/craniodorsal)
- Luxation of the ileosacral joint
- Hip dysplasia (HD)
- Tumour
- Osteomyelitis
- Arthritis/arthrosis (coxarthrosis)
- Deformations (Coxa valga/vara)
- Aseptic femoral head necrosis (Legg-Calve-Perthes disease)
- Osteochondrosis dissecans (OCD)

Pelvis
- Fracture
- Tumour

Endoscopy: Arthroscopy

Indication

- Joint disease of unknown origin
- Biopsy and surgery

Arthroscopy

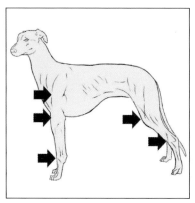

Fig 9.198 Suitable joints for arthroscopy

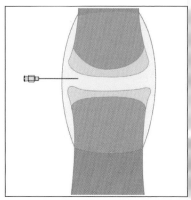

Fig 9.199 Flushing channel access: puncture with a hypodermic needle

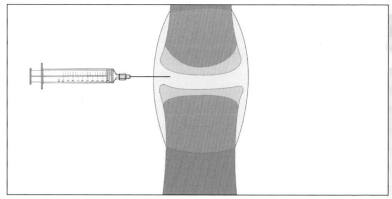

Fig 9.200 Flushing channel access: injection of physiological sterile saline for the expansion of the joint capsule

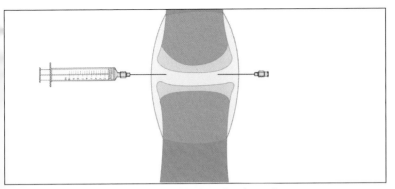

Fig 9.201 Endoscopy channel: puncture with a hypodermic needle

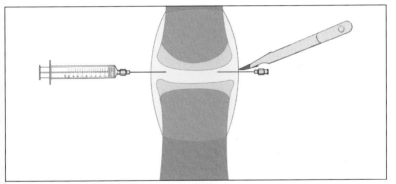

Fig 9.202 Endoscopy channel: enlargement of the access point with a scalpel blade

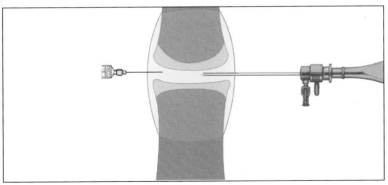

Fig 9.203 Endoscopy channel: insertion of the shaft and trocar

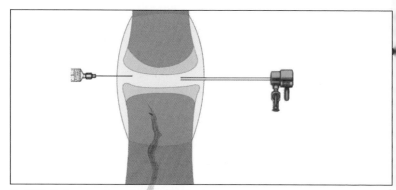

Fig 9.204 Endoscopy channel: removal of the trocar

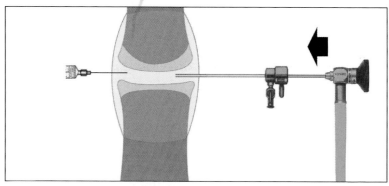

Fig 9.205 Endoscopy channel: insertion of the endoscope into the shaft

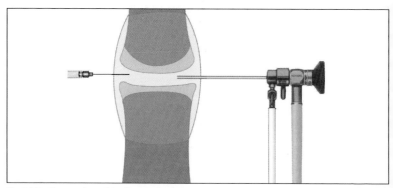

Fig 9.206 Connection of the flushing hoses

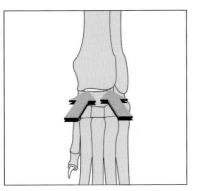

Fig 9.207 Access to the carpal joint

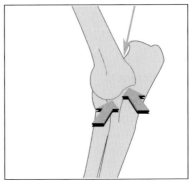

Fig 9.208 Access to the elbow joint

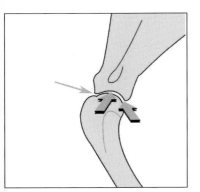

Fig 9.209 Access to the shoulder joint

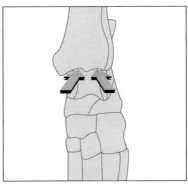

Fig 9.210 Access to the tarsal joint
(dorsal/cranial)

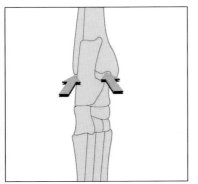

Fig 9.211 Access to the tarsal joint
(ventral/caudal)

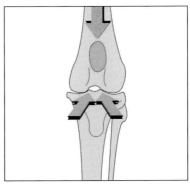

Fig 9.212 Access to the knee joint

Method

- **Preparation**
  - General anaesthesia
  - Lateral recumbency/sternal/prone position
  - Clip fur/disinfect skin

- **Technique**

  Flushing channel access
  - Puncture the joint with a hypodermic needle (20–22 G)
  - Attach a 2ml syringe
  - Inject physiological sterile saline for the expansion of the joint capsule

  Endoscopy channel access
  - Puncture the joint with a hypodermic needle (20–22 G)
  - Enlarge the access point with a scalpel blade
  - Remove the hypodermic needle
  - Insert the endoscope shaft and trocar
  - Remove the trocar
  - Insert the endoscope into the shaft
  - Connect the flushing hoses (in/outlet) (flush with saline)

Complications

- Infection
- Arthrosis

Ultrasound Examination

Indication

• Muscle, tendon or joint disease of unknown origin

Ultrasound Examination

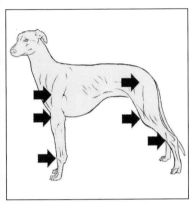

Fig 9.213 Suitable joints for an ultrasound examination

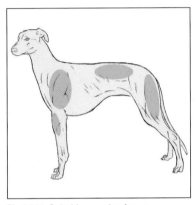

Fig 9.214 Suitable muscles for an ultrasound examination

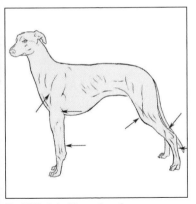

Fig 9.215 Suitable tendons for an ultrasound examination

Joint Biopsy

Indication

- Chronic joint disease of unknown origin
- Suspected tumour

Joint Biopsy

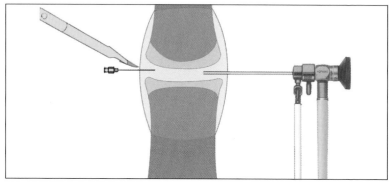

Fig 9.216 Biopsy channel access: joint puncture with a hypodermic needle and expansion of the access point with a scalpel blade

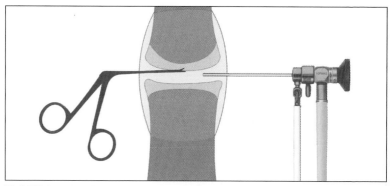

Fig 9.217 Insertion of a biopsy forceps and biopsy under endoscopic visual control

Bone Marrow Biopsy

Indication

- Non–regenerative anaemia
- Suspected tumour

Bone Marrow Biopsy (Aspiration Biopsy)

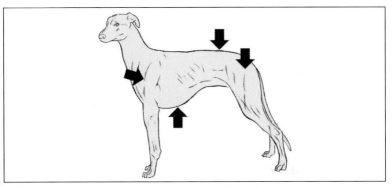

Fig 9.218 Suitable puncture sites for a bone marrow biopsy in the dog

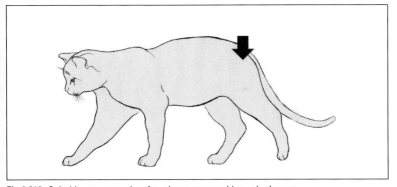

Fig 9.219 Suitable puncture sites for a bone marrow biopsy in the cat

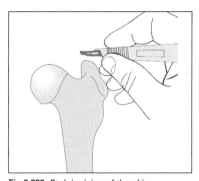

Fig 9.220 Stab incision of the skin

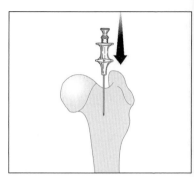

Fig 9.221 Drilling movements with the biopsy needle into the bone marrow

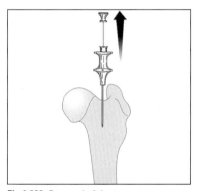

Fig 9.222 Removal of the trocar

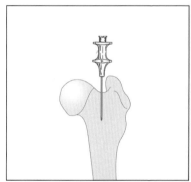

Fig 9.223 Position of the biopsy needle in the bone marrow

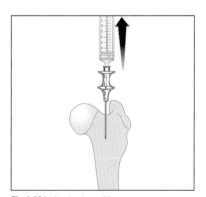

Fig 9.224 Aspiration of bone marrow

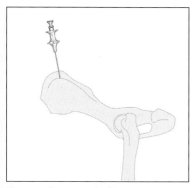

Fig 9.225 Access to the iliac wing

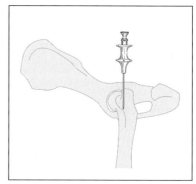

Fig 9.226 Access to the femur

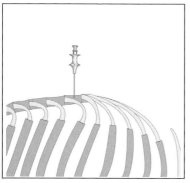

Fig 9.227 Access to the sternum

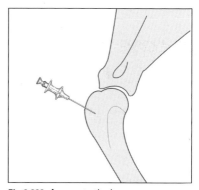

Fig 9.228 Access to the humerus

Bone Marrow Biopsy (Punch Biopsy)

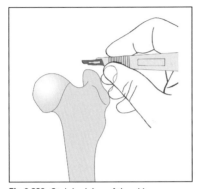

Fig 9.229 Stab incision of the skin

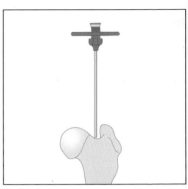

Fig 9.230 Drilling movements of the biopsy needle into the bone marrow

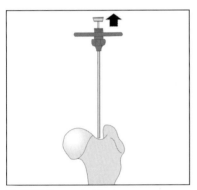

Fig 9.231 Removal of the trocar

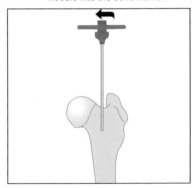

Fig 9.232 Rotation and removal of the biopsy needle

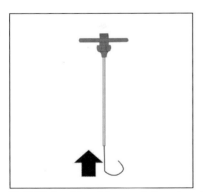

Fig 9.233 Expulsion of the sample from the biopsy needle

Bone Biopsy

Indication

• Bone disease of unknown origin (osteomyelitis, tumour)

Bone Biopsy

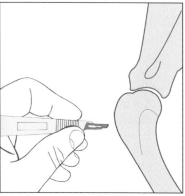

Fig 9.234 Stab incision of the skin

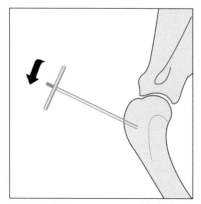

Fig 9.235 Drilling movements with the bone biopsy needle

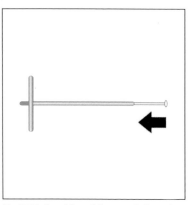

Fig 9.236 Expulsion of the sample from the needle core

Method

- **Preparation**
  - Sedation/general anaesthesia
  - Clip fur/disinfect skin

- **Technique**
  - Joint biopsy
  - Endoscopy channel access
  - Biopsy channel access:
    - Puncture the joint with a hypodermic needle, expand the access point with a scalpel blade
  - Insert the biopsy forceps into the biopsy channel
  - Take the biopsy under endoscopic visual control

Bone marrow biopsy (aspiration biopsy)

- Dog: crista iliaca (iliac wing), trochanteric fossa of the femur, sternum, major tubercle of the humerus
- Cat: trochanteric fossa of the femur
- Make a stab incision of the skin
- Perform drilling movements with the puncture cannula and stylet (Rosenthal-cannula 16/18 G, Illinois-needle into the bone marrow) (Klima needle and Jamshidi needle are also used)
- Remove the stylet
- Attach a 10 or 20ml syringe and aspirate the bone marrow until it is visible in the syringe

Bone marrow biopsy (punch biopsy)

- Dog: trochanteric fossa of the femur, major tubercle of the humerus
- Cat: trochanteric fossa of the femur
- Make a stab incision of the skin
- Perform drilling movements with the puncture cannula and stylet (Jamshidi needle) into the bone marrow
- Remove the stylet
- Advance the needle for about 1–2cm
- Twist the needle repeatedly around the longitudinal axis
- Remove the needle and obtained sample

Bone biopsy

- Localise the biopsy area with previously taken X-rays
- Make a stab incision of the skin
- Perform drilling movements with the puncture cannula without the stylet (Jamshidi needle) through the cortex of the bone into the bone marrow
- Remove the cannula with a core of bone

Complications

- Haemorrhage
- Pathological fracture
- Infection

Arthrocentesis

Indication

- Arthritis of unknown origin (cytology, bacterial examination)
- Administration of medicines/radiographic contrast media

Arthrocentesis

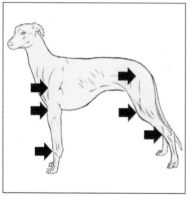

Fig 9.237 Suitable puncture sites in the dog

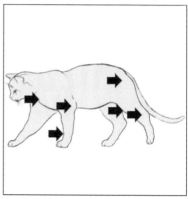

Fig 9.238 Suitable puncture sites in the cat

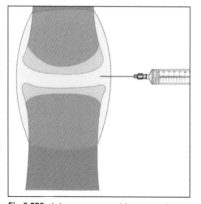

Fig 9.239 Joint puncture with an attached syringe

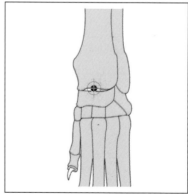

Fig 9.240 Access to the carpal joint

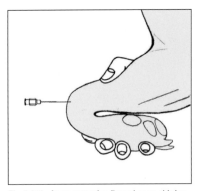

Fig 9.241 Access to the flexed carpal joint

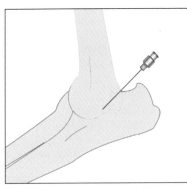

Fig 9.242 Access to the elbow joint

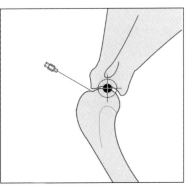

Fig 9.243 Access to the shoulder joint

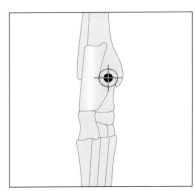

Fig 9.244 Access to the tarsal joint

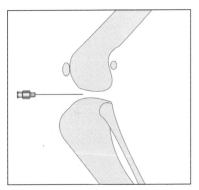

Fig 9.245 Access to the knee joint

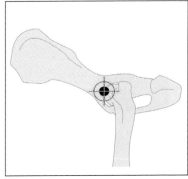

Fig 9.246 Access to the hip joint

Method

- **Preparation**
  - Sedation
  - Partial flexion of the joints
  - Clip fur/disinfect skin

- **Technique**
  - Palpate the joint effusion
  - Puncture the joint with a hypodermic needle and attached syringe (22 G)
  - Aspirate (c. 0.5ml)

Complications

- Infection
- Haemorrhage

Further Orthopaedic Examination Methods

- Laboratory tests
- Muscle biopsy
- Nerve biopsy
- Computer tomography (CT)
- Magnetic resonance tomography (MRT)
- Scintigraphy

10 Neurological Examination Methods

Case History

Principal Symptoms

- Behavioural disorder
- Coma
- Syncope
- Convulsions
- Tremor
- Urinary incontinence/retention
- Paresis/paralysis
- Head tilt
- Hyperaesthesia
- Loss of eyesight/blindness
- Nystagmus
- Strabismus
- Anisocoria
- Vomitus
- Polydipsia
- Hearing loss/deafness
- Opisthotonus
- Torticollis
- Ataxia
- Dysphagia
- Narcolepsy/catalepsy/-plexy
- Tetany
- Schiff-Sherrington syndrome

Inspection

Indication

• Part of the general examination

Inspection

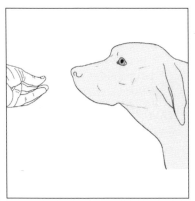

Fig 10.1 Mentation and behaviour

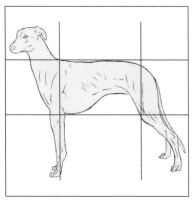

Fig 10.2 Body posture/limb position and posture

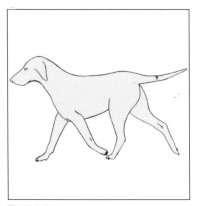

Fig 10.3 Gait

Method

- **Technique**
  - Observation at rest

- **Evaluation criteria**
  - Mentation, behaviour, body posture,
  - Limb position and posture

Findings

- **Physiological**
  - Bright and alert, appropriate to the environment
  - Symmetric and controlled body posture and limb position
  - Coordinated movements

- **Pathological**

  Mentation
  - Depression/lethargy/apathy
  - Stupor/coma

  Behaviour
  - Disorientation
  - Compulsion
  - Aggression
  - Hyperactivity
  - Fearfulness
  - Lethargy/apathy
  - Seizures/tremor
  - Ataxia

Body posture/limb position
- Head tilt
- Lowering of the head
- Torticollis
- Opisthotonus
- Schiff-Sherrington syndrome
- Curved back
- Hyperextension/-flexion
- Wide-based stance
- Knuckling of the paw
- Extensor hypertonia/decerebration syndrome
- Scuffed claws

Gait
- Ataxia
- Lameness/paralysis
- Circling
- Hypermetria

Palpation

Indication

- Part of the general examination

Palpation

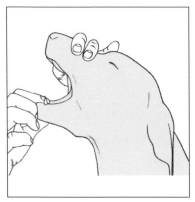

Fig 10.4 Function test of the mandible

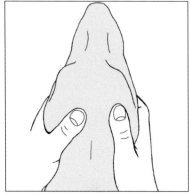

Fig 10.5 Palpation of the head muscles

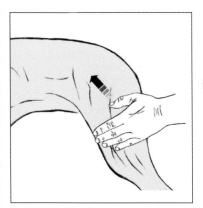

Fig 10.6 Comparative palpation of the musculature

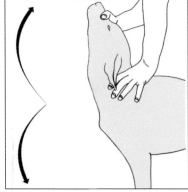

Fig 10.7 Flexion and extension of the cervical spine

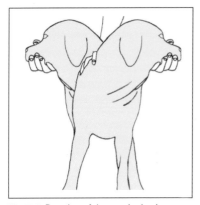

Fig 10.8 Rotation of the cervical spine

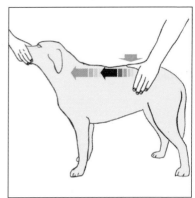

Fig 10.9 Palpation of the spine

Method

- **Evaluation criteria**
  - Size, shape, symmetry, consistency, temperature, stability, painfulness, crepitus

- **Technique**

  Head
  - Palpation of the head muscles
  - Opening and closure of the mandible (jaw occlusion)

  Cervical spine
  - Extension/flexion and rotation towards both sides

  Thoracic and lumbar spine
  - Pressure palpation of each vertebra from caudal towards cranial

Findings

- **Physiological**
  - Nothing abnormal to detect (NAD)

- **Pathological**

  Spine
  - Spinal lesion/meningitis/meningoencephalitis

  Musculature
  - Atrophy
  - Changes of the muscle tone

Postural Responses

Indication

- Neurological examination method

Postural Responses

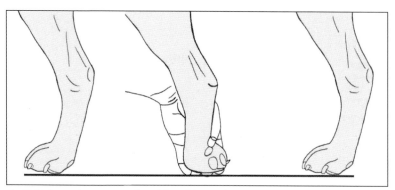

Fig 10.10 Correction response (knuckling of the paw)

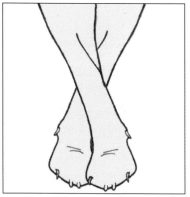

Fig 10.11 Correction response (crossing of the limbs)

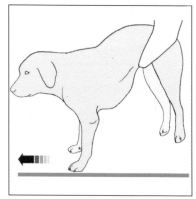

Fig 10.12 Wheelbarrowing response (visual)

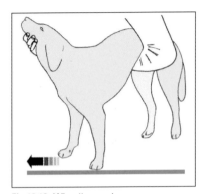

Fig 10.13 Wheelbarrowing response (tactile)

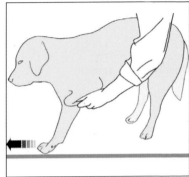

Fig 10.14 Hopping response (straight ahead)

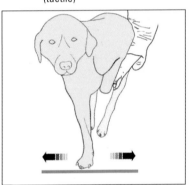

Fig 10.15 Side stepping response (lateral)

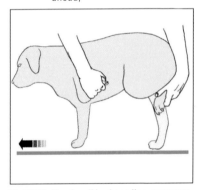

Fig 10.16 Hemi walking/standing response

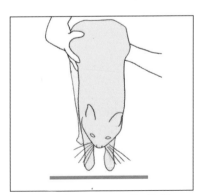

Fig 10.17 Righting response (forelimb)

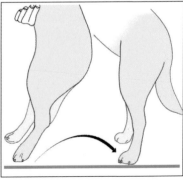

Fig 10.18 Righting response (hind limb)

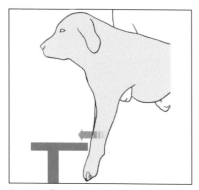

Fig 10.19 Table edge response/placing response (visual)

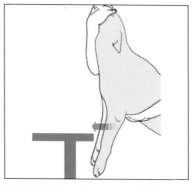

Fig 10.20 Table edge response/placing response (tactile)

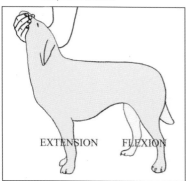

Fig 10.21 Tonic neck reaction (extension of the head)

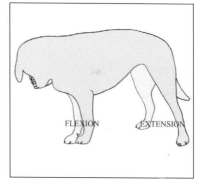

Fig 10.22 Tonic neck reaction (flexion of the head)

Method

- **Technique**

    Correction responses
    - Place all paws one after the other into the knuckling position
    - Cross over the fore and hind limb pairs

    Wheelbarrowing responses
    - Visual: lift the caudal body half while pushing the body forwards/lateral
    - Tactile: lift the caudal body half while elevating the head and push the body forwards/lateral

Hopping response
– Lift three limbs at a time and push the body forwards/lateral

Hemi walking/standing
– Lift one ipsilateral pair of limbs while pushing the body forwards/lateral

Righting response
– Forelimbs: suspend the body by the pelvis and place the animal onto its forelimbs
– Hind limbs: suspend the body by the thorax and place the animal onto its hind limbs

Table edge response/placing response
– Visual: approach the table edge with the forelimbs
– Tactile: approach the table edge with the forelimbs while covering the eyes

Tonic neck reaction
– Extend/flex the neck

Findings

- **Physiological**

Correction response
– Immediate correction of the paw into the physiological position

Wheelbarrowing response
– Coordinated sequence of steps

Hopping response
– Coordinated hopping

Hemi walking/standing response
– Coordinated hopping

Righting response
– Forelimb: the patient lifts the head and extends the forelimb
– Hind limb: the patient extends the hind limb and steps backwards once ground contact is made

Table edge response/placing response
– The patient places the feet onto the table surface in a coordinated manner

Tonic neck reaction
- Extension of the head: the patient extends the forelimbs and flexes the hind limbs
- Flexion of the head: the patient flexes the forelimbs and extends the hind limbs

- **Pathological**

Correction responses
- Delayed response, correction is absent (paresis)

Wheelbarrowing response
- Delayed, uncoordinated, absent sequence of steps (lesion of the cervical spine, brain stem or cerebral cortex)
- Increased/exaggerated sequence of steps/hypermetria (cerebellar lesion)

Hopping response
- Absence in the forelimbs (lesion of the cervical spine, brain stem or cerebral cortex)
- Absence in the hind limbs (lesion of the lumbar spine, brain stem or cerebral cortex)
- Increased/exaggerated sequence of steps/hypermetria (cerebellar lesion)

Hemi walking/standing
- Absence in one ipsilateral limb pair (lesion of the cerebral cortex in the contralateral side)

Righting response
- Absence (lesions of the spinal cord, brain stem or cerebral cortex)
- Increased/exaggerated sequence of steps/hypermetria (lesion of the vestibular system or cerebellum)

Table-edge response/placing response
- Visual absence
- Tactile absence (disorder of deep sensitivity)
- Tonic neck reaction
- Absences (lesion of the cervical spine, brain stem or cerebral cortex)
- Increased/exaggerated sequence of steps/hypermetria (cerebellar lesion)

Spinal Reflexes

Indication

- Neurological examination

Spinal Reflexes

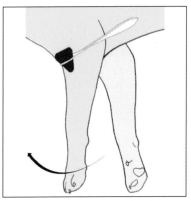

Fig 10.23 Extensor carpi radialis reflex

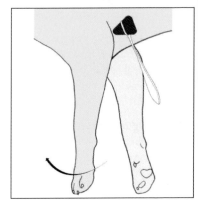

Fig 10.24 Triceps reflex

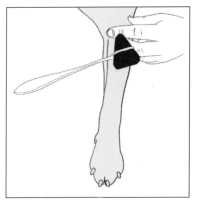

Fig 10.25 Bicipital reflex

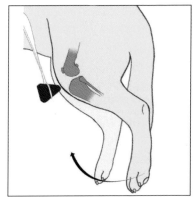

Fig 10.26 Patellar reflex

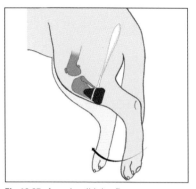

Fig 10.27 Anterior tibial reflex

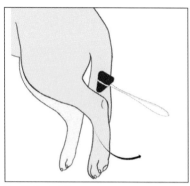

Fig 10.28 Achilles tendon reflex

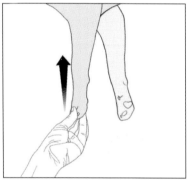

Fig 10.29 Withdrawal reflex (flexor reflex)

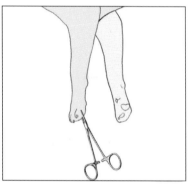

Fig 10.30 Withdrawal reflex (flexor reflex)

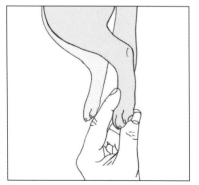

Fig 10.31 Withdrawal reflex (extensor reflex)

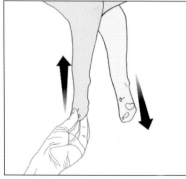

Fig 10.32 Pathological withdrawal reflex (crossed extensor reflex)

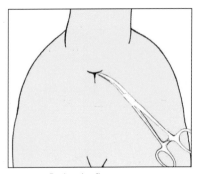

Fig 10.33 Perineal reflex

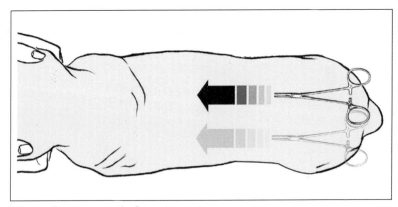

Fig 10.34 Cutaneous trunci reflex

Method

- **Technique**

  ### Extensor-carpi-radialis reflex
  – Lift the flexed elbow, tap the radial extensor of the carpus muscle

  ### Triceps reflex
  – Lift the flexed elbow
  – Tap the triceps tendon cranial of the olecranon

Bicipital reflex
– Place and tap the biceps muscle with your forefinger while the elbow is extended

Patellar reflex/quadriceps reflex
– Lift the knee while the patient is in lateral recumbency and tap the patellar tendon

Anterior tibial reflex
– Tap the cranial tibial muscle distally/laterally of the knee joint

Achilles tendon reflex/gastrocnemius reflex
– Lift the knee joint and tap the Achilles tendon cranial of the calcaneum

Withdrawal reflex (flexor reflex)
– Pinch the interdigital skin, digits and pads

Withdrawal reflex (extensor reflex)
– Massage the interdigital skin

Pathological withdrawal reflex (crossed extensor reflex)
– Pinch the interdigital skin, digits and pads
– Observe the contralateral limb

Perineal reflex
– Touch/pinch the skin of the perineum, vulva and prepuce

Cutaneous trunci reflex
– Touch/pinch the skin of the paravertebral dorsal region from caudal towards cranial (between L4 and C8)

Findings

• **Physiological**

Extensor-carpi-radialis reflex
– Extension of the carpal joint

Triceps reflex
– Extension of the elbow joint

Biceps reflex
– Flexion of the elbow joint

Patellar reflex/quadriceps reflex
– Extension of the knee joint

Anterior tibial reflex
– Extension of the knee joint

Achilles tendon reflex/gastrocneumius reflex
– Extension of the tarsal joint

Withdrawal reflex (flexor reflex)
– Withdrawal of the limb

Withdrawal reflex (extensor reflex)
– Extension of the limb

Perineal reflex
– Contraction of the anal sphincter and flexion of the tail

Cutaneous trunci reflex
– Contraction of the skin muscles

• **Pathological**

Extensor-carpi-radialis reflex
– Absence (lesion of the radial nerve, spinal lesion C7–T2)
– Hyperreflexia (spinal lesion cranial of C7)

Triceps reflex
– Absence (lesion of the radial nerve, spinal lesion C7–T2)
– Hyperreflexia (spinal lesion cranial of C7)

Bicipital reflex
– Absence (lesion of the musculocutaneus nerve, spinal lesion C6–C7)
– Hyperreflexia (spinal lesion cranial of C6)

Patellar reflex/quadriceps reflex
– Absence (lesion of the femoral nerve, spinal lesion L4–L5)
– Hyperreflexia (chronic spinal lesion cranial of L4 with loss of inhibition)

Tibialis anterior reflex
– Absence (lesion of the sciatic nerve, spinal lesion L6–S2)
– Hyperreflexia (spinal lesion cranial of L6)

Achilles tendon reflex/gastrocneumius reflex
– Absence (lesion of the sciatic nerve, spinal lesion L6–S2)
– Hyperreflexia (spinal lesion cranial of L6)

Withdrawal reflex (flexor reflex)
- Absence (spinal lesion C6–T1 or rather L4–S1)
- Hyperreflexia (spinal lesion cranial of C6 or rather L4)

Withdrawal reflex (extensor reflex)
- Absence (spinal lesion C6–T1 or rather L4–S1, lesion of the sciatic nerve)
- Hyperreflexia (spinal lesion cranial of C6 or rather L4)

Pathological withdrawal reflex (crossed extensor reflex)
- Spinal lesion cranial of C6 or rather L4

Perineal reflex
- Absence (pudendal nerve, spinal lesion S1–S3)

Cutaneous trunci reflex
- Absence (spinal lesion cranial of the absence C8–L4)

Cranial Nerves

Indication

- Neurological examination

Cranial Nerves

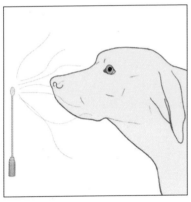

Fig 10.35 Olfactory test

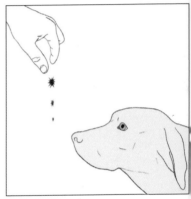

Fig 10.36 Sight test/following movement test

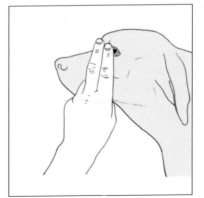

Fig 10.37 Menace response

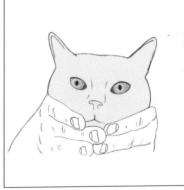

Fig 10.38 Ocular/bulbus and pupillary position

Cranial Nerve Function Test

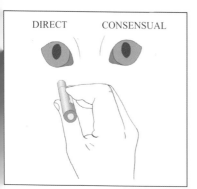

Fig 10.39 Pupillary light reflex

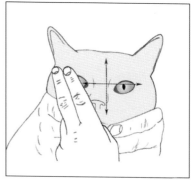

Fig 10.40 Eye mobility and movements

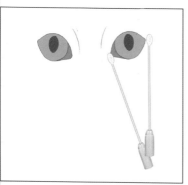

Fig 10.41 Palpebral reflex (blink reflex)

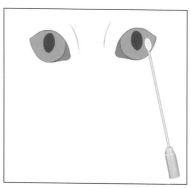

Fig 10.42 Corneal reflex (blink reflex)

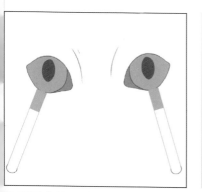

Fig 10.43 Schirmer tear test

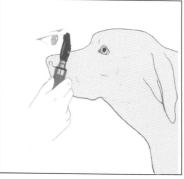

Fig 10.44 Ophthalmoscopy/examination of the ocular fundus

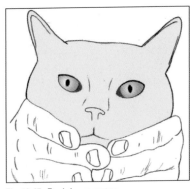

Fig 10.45 Facial symmetry

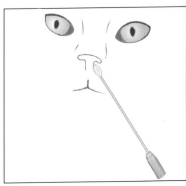

Fig 10.46 Nasal sensitivity

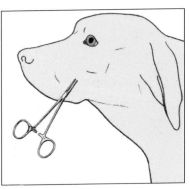

Fig 10.47 Facial sensitivity

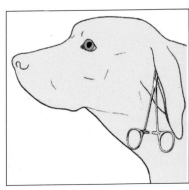

Fig 10.48 Ear mobility

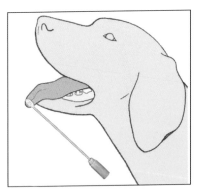

Fig 10.49 Taste test (atropine test)

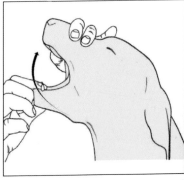

Fig 10.50 Jaw occlusion

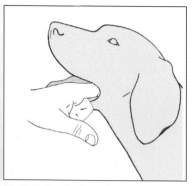

Fig 10.51 Swallowing reflex

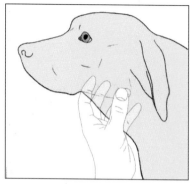

Fig 10.52 Swallowing/gag reflex

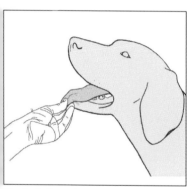

Fig 10.53 Glossal mobility

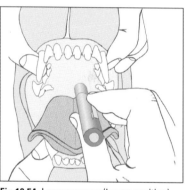

Fig 10.54 Laryngoscopy (larynx position)

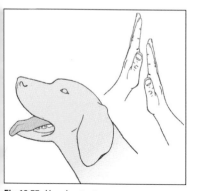

Fig 10.55 Hearing test

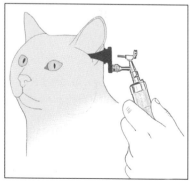

Fig 10.56 Otoscopy

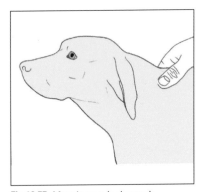

Fig 10.57 Muscle tone in the neck musculature

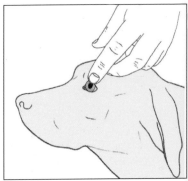

Fig 10.58 Oculo-cardial reflex (eyeball compression-auscultation)

Method

- **Technique**

    Olfactory test
    – Offer some cotton wool soaked in alcohol

    Sight test/following movement test
    – Drop some cotton wool within the visual field

    Menace response
    – Make fast movements with your finger towards the eye

    Eye/globe position
    – Inspect and compare the eyes with each other

    Pupillary position
    – Inspect and compare the eyes with each other

    Pupillary light reflex (PLR)
    – Direct: pupillary reaction in the lit eye (swinging movements with the light)
    – Consensual: pupillary reaction in the non-lit eye

    Eye mobility
    – The eyes are following the finger in all directions

Eye movements
- Observe spontaneous eye movements and establish if these can be triggered (nystagmus)

Palpebral reflex
- Touch the eyelids with a cotton bud

Corneal reflex
- Touch the cornea with a cotton bud

Schirmer tear test
- Insert the Schirmer test strips into the lower lateral conjunctiva, place the notch at the edge of the lid
- Hold both eyelids shut
- Take the reading of the tear production after 1 min

Ophthalmoscopy
- Examine the ocular fundus

Facial symmetry
- Inspect

Nasal sensitivity
- Pinch the nasal plane region slightly with a pair of forceps

Facial sensitivity
- Pinch the facial region slightly with a pair of forceps

Aural mobility
- Touch the pinna with a finger or pair of forceps

Taste test
- Dab the tip of the tongue with a swab soaked in atropine

Jaw occlusion
- Open and close the mandible

Swallowing reflex
- Insert a finger into the pharynx
- Palpate the larynx externally

Glossal mobility
- (Attempt to) grasp the tongue

Laryngoscope
- Inspect the larynx

Hearing test
– Create a sound (clapping, whistling etc.) outside the patient's field of vision

Otoscopy
– Examine the external ear canal/tympanic membrane

Muscle tone of the neck musculature
– Palpate the neck muscles (trapezius muscle, brachiocephalic muscle, sternocephalic muscle)

Oculo-cardial reflex
– Auscultate the heart before and after applying pressure on the bulbus

Findings

- **Physiological**

  ### Olfactory test
  – Aversion

  ### Sight test/following movement test
  – The patient looks up and follows the movement of the cotton wool

  ### Menace response
  – Blink

  ### Eye/globe position
  – Physiological

  ### Pupillary position
  – Symmetric, appropriate for the situation

  ### Pupillary light reflex (PLR)
  – Direct: miosis
  – Consensual: miosis

  ### Eye mobility
  – The eyes follow the movements of the finger

  ### Eye movements
  – No nystagmus

  ### Palpebral reflex
  – Blink

Corneal reflex
- Blink

Schirmer tear test
- Normal values: dog (21.9 ± 4.0 mm), cat (20.2 ± 4.5 mm)

Ophthalmoscopy
- Physiological ocular fundus

Facial symmetry
- Symmetric

Nasal sensitivity
- Nasal twitch

Facial sensitivity
- Skin twitches

Aural mobility
- Ear movement

Taste test
- Aversion

Jaw occlusion
- Physiological

Swallowing reflex
- Physiological

Glossal mobility
- Tongue movement

Laryngoscopy
- Symmetrical larynx

Hearing test
- Ear/pinnal movements

Otoscopy
- Physiological

Muscle tone of the neck musculature
- Physiological

Oculo-cardial reflex
- Bradycardia

- **Pathological**

  Olfactory test
  – Absence (CN I, olfactory nerve)

  Sight test/following movement test
  – Absence (CN II, optic nerve, retina, optic tracts, cerebral cortex)

  Menace response
  – Absence (CN II, optic nerve; CN VII, facial nerve)

  Eye/bulbus position
  – Absence (CN III, oculomotor nerve; IV, trochlear nerve; VI, abducent nerve, mesencephalon, medulla oblongata)
  – Exophthalmus
  – Enophthalmus

  Pupillary position
  – Miosis
  – Mydriasis
  – Anisocoria (sympathetic nerve, parasympathetic nerve)
  – Strabismus (CN III, oculmotor nerve; IV, trochlear nerve; VI, abducent nerve)

  Pupillary light reflex
  – Direct: absence (lesion of the afferent and/or efferent nerves of the stimulated eye)
  – Consensual: absence (lesion of the afferent nerves of the stimulated eye and/or efferent nerves of the contralateral eye)

  Eye mobility
  – Absence (CN II, III, IV, VI)

  Eye movements
  – Horizontal nystagmus (peripheral or central vestibular disorder)
  – Vertical nystagmus (central vestibular disorder)

  Palpebral reflex
  – Absence (CN V, trigeminal nerve; VII, facial nerve)

  Corneal reflex
  – Absence (CN V, VII)

  Schirmer tear test
  – Absence (CN VII, keratoconjunctivitis sicca)

Ophthalmoscopy
- Lesion of the optical nerve or retinal lesion

Facial symmetry
- Absence (CN VII)

Nasal sensitivity
- Absence (CN V, VII)

Facial sensitivity
- Absence (CN V, VII)

Aural mobility
- Absence (CN VII)

Taste test
- Absence (CN VII)

Jaw occlusion
- Absence (CN V)

Swallowing reflex
- Absence (CN IX, glossopharyngeal nerve; X, vagus nerve)

Glossal mobility
- Absence (CN XII, hypoglossal nerve)

Laryngoscopy
- Laryngeal paralysis (CN X, XI-spinal accessory nerve)

Hearing test
- Absence (CN VIII)

Otoscopy
- Otitis externa/media, tumour

Muscle tone of the neck musculature
- Atrophy (CN XI)

Oculo-cardial reflex
- Absence (CN V, X)

Sensory Perception

Indication

- Neurological examination

Sensory Perception: Innervation Areas/Dermatomes

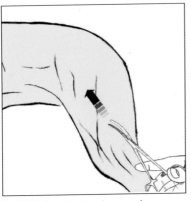

Fig 10.59 Superficial pain sensation

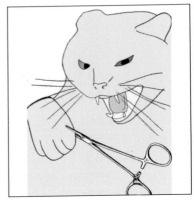

Fig 10.60 Deep pain sensation

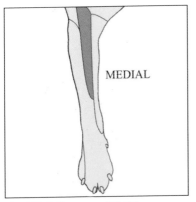

MEDIAL

Fig 10.61 Axillary nerve (C6–C8)

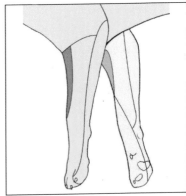

Fig 10.62 Axillary nerve (C6–C8)

Sensory Perception: Innervation Areas/Dermatomes (Forelimb)

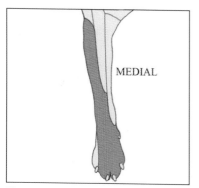

Fig 10.63 Radial nerve (C7–T2)

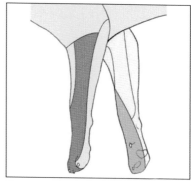

Fig 10.64 Radial nerve (C7–T2)

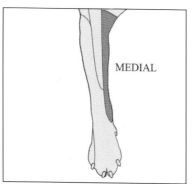

Fig 10.65 Musculocutaneos nerve (C6–C8)

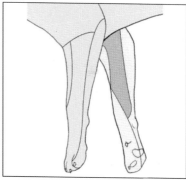

Fig 10.66 Musculocutaneos nerve (C6–C8)

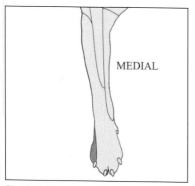

Fig 10.67 Ulnar nerve (C8–T2)

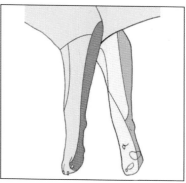

Fig 10.68 Ulnar nerve (C8–T2)

Sensory Perception: Innervation Areas/Dermatomes (Hind Limb)

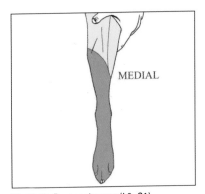

Fig 10.69 Peroneal nerve (L6–S1)

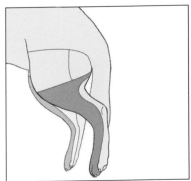

Fig 10.70 Peroneal nerve (L6–S1)

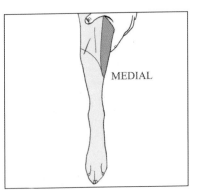

Fig 10.71 Sapheneous nerve (L4–L5)

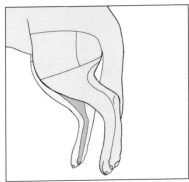

Fig 10.72 Sapheneous nerve (L4–L5)

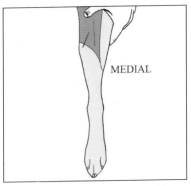

Fig 10.73 Lateral cutaneous nerve of the thigh (L7–S2)

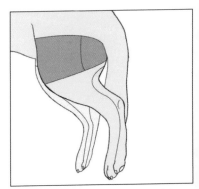

Fig 10.74 Lateral cutaneous nerve of the thigh (L7–S2)

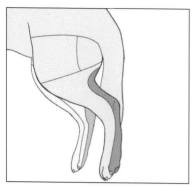

Fig 10.75 Tibial nerve (L6–S1)

Method

- **Technique**
    - Superficial pain sensation: pinch the skin with a pair of artery forceps, needle or pencil
    - Deep pain sensation: pinch the digits/periosteum with a pair of artery forceps

Findings

- **Physiological**
    - Superficial pain sensation: the skin muscles twitch
    - Deep pain sensation: pain reaction

- **Pathological**
    - Peripheral nerve lesion
    - Spinal lesion
    - Central lesion

Plain X-Ray Study

Indication

- Diseases of the vertebral spine/spinal cord, e.g., vestibular dysfunctions, dysphagia, vision disorders

X-Ray Study: Head

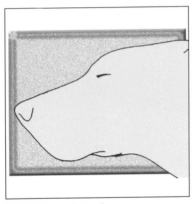

Fig 10.76 Head (lateral)

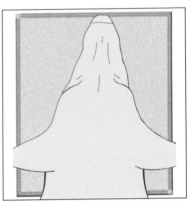

Fig 10.77 Head (dorsoventral)

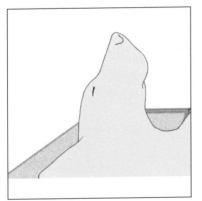

Fig 10.78 Sinus view (frontal)

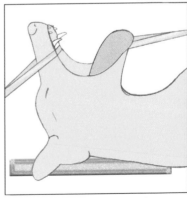

Fig 10.79 Bullar view/Dens-axis view

X-Ray Study: Spine

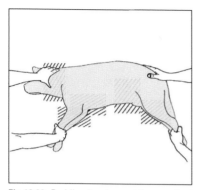

Fig 10.80 Padding for views of the vertebral spine

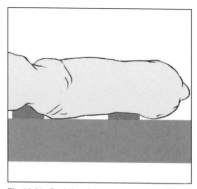

Fig 10.81 Padding for views of the vertebral spine

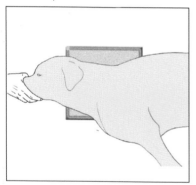

Fig 10.82 Cervical spine (lateral)

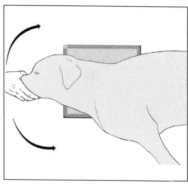

Fig 10.83 Cervical spine, tension views (lateral)

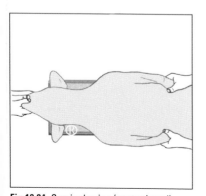

Fig 10.84 Cervical spine (ventrodorsal)

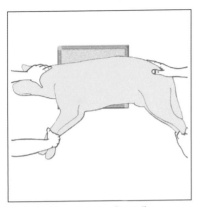

Fig 10.85 Thoracic spine (lateral)

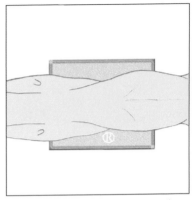

Fig 10.86 Thoracic spine (ventrodorsal)

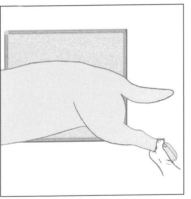

Fig 10.87 Lumbar spine/cauda equina (lateral)

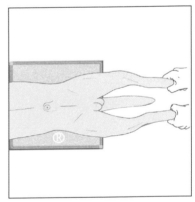

Fig 10.88 Lumbar spine/cauda equina (ventrodorsal)

Method

- **Technique**
  - Cervical spine: central beam C3–C4
  - Thoracic spine: central beam T6–7
  - Lumbar spine: central beam L4–5
  - Cauda equina: central beam L7–S1
  - Tension views (Wobbler syndrome)

Findings

- **Physiological**
  - Nothing abnormal to detect (NAD)

- **Pathological**

  Head
  - Tumour
  - Abscess
  - Sinusitis
  - Otitis media/tympanic bulla
  - Radiopaque foreign body

  Cervical spine
  - Vertebral fracture/Dens-axis fracture
  - Luxation
  - Atlantoaxial subluxation
  - Wobbler syndrome
  - Intervertebral disc prolapse (collapsed intervertebral disc space)
  - Discospondylitis/osteomyelitis
  - Spondylosis deformans
  - Tumour

  Thoracic-/lumbar spine
  - Vertebral fracture
  - Luxation
  - Intervertebral disc prolapse
  - Discospondylitis/osteomyelitis
  - Spondylosis deformans
  - Tumour
  - Lumbosacral stenosis (cauda-equina syndrome)
  - Osteoporosis/-petrosis/hypervitaminosis A
  - Vertebral deformities

Myelography

Indication

- Paresis/paralysis

Method

- **Preparation**
  - General anaesthesia (avoid drugs which may precipitate convulsions like ketamine)
  - Lateral recumbency (90° angle of the head)
  - Clip fur/disinfect skin

- **Technique**

  Cisternal myelography
  - Perform a fluid puncture of the cerebellomedullary cistern in the dorsal subarachnoid space
  - Remove the fluid (let it drip off 0.5–2.0ml)
  - Slowly inject some bodywarm contrast media via fluoroscopy (C-arch) (0.3–0.5ml/kg)
  - Contrast media: Iopamidol
  - Iohexol (Omnipaque®), Iotrolan (Isovist®)
  - Remove the spinal needle
  - X-ray views: cervical/thoracic spine: (l + vd) immediately, consider repeating after elevation of the head for 1–2 mins

  Lumbar myelography
  - Perform a fluid puncture in the ventral subarachnoid space between L5–6 (large dogs), L6–7 (small dogs/cats)
  - Remove the fluid (wait for it to drip passively into a tube) (0.5–2.0ml)
  - Slowly inject bodywarm contrast medium via fluoroscopy (C-arch) (0.3–0.5ml/kg)
  - Contrast media: Iopamidol/Iohexol (Omnipaque®)/Iotrolan (Isovist®)
  - Remove the spinal needle
  - X-ray views: lumbar/thoracic spine: (l + vd) immediately, consider repeating after elevation of the pelvis for 1–2 min

Findings

- **Physiological**
    - Unimpeded flow of the contrast medium

- **Pathological**
    - Contrast medium flow impediment (space occupying lesion)

Extradural
- Intervertebral disc prolapse
- Vertebral fracture/luxation
- Tumour
- Abscess
- Haematoma
- Oedema

Intradural/extramedullary
- Tumour
- Haematoma
- Arachnoid cyst
- Meningocele

Intramedullary
- Tumour
- Oedema
- Haemorrhage/haematoma
- Myelomalacia

Complications

- Haemorrhage
- Convulsions
- Injury of the spinal cord
- Infection
- Respiratory arrest
- Brain herniation (in case of increased intracranial pressure)

Cerebrospinal Fluid Puncture/CSF Tap

Indication

- CNS disease of unknown origin
- Myelography

Cerebrospinal Fluid Puncture/CSF Tap

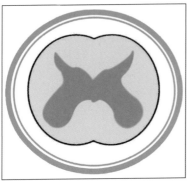

Fig 10.89 Cross section of the spinal cord

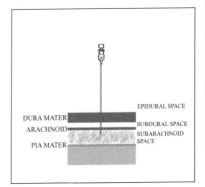

Fig 10.90 Fluid puncture in the dorsal subarachnoid space

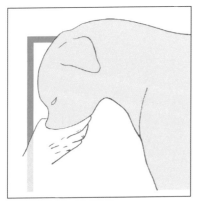

Fig 10.91 90° angulation of the head (cisternal puncture)

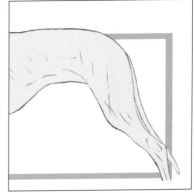

Fig 10.92 Position for a lumbar puncture

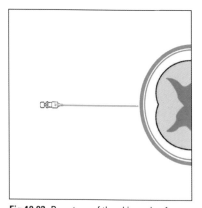

Fig 10.93 Puncture of the skin and soft tissues

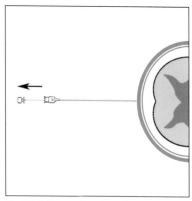

Fig 10.94 Removal of the stylet

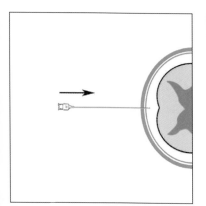

Fig 10.95 Puncture of the dura mater/arachnoid

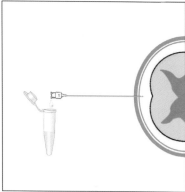

Fig 10.96 Collection of the fluid (subarachnoid space)

Fluid Puncture: Cisternal

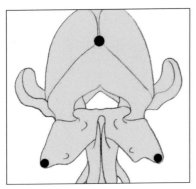

Fig 10.97 Palpation: occipital protuberance/wing of the atlas

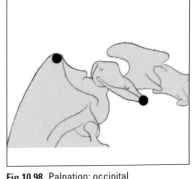

Fig 10.98 Palpation: occipital protuberance/wing of the atlas

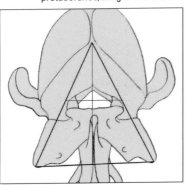

Fig 10.99 Puncture site, method 1: in the centre of the triangle

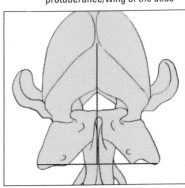

Fig 10.100 Puncture site, method 2: in the middle of the connection line

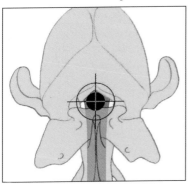

Fig 10.101 Puncture site for the cisternal fluid puncture

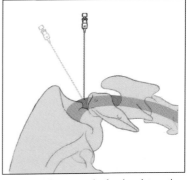

Fig 10.102 Puncture site for the cisternal fluid puncture

Fluid Puncture: Lumbar

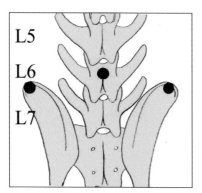

Fig 10.103 Palpation: spinous process L6/iliac wing

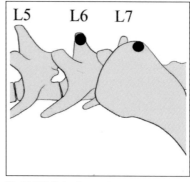

Fig 10.104 Palpation: spinous process L6/iliac wing

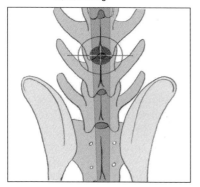

Fig 10.105 Puncture site for the lumbar fluid puncture

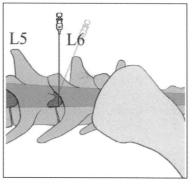

Fig 10.106 Puncture site for the lumbar fluid puncture (dog)

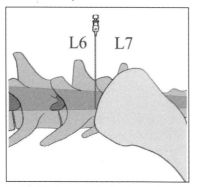

Fig 10.107 Puncture site for the lumbar fluid puncture (cat)

Method

- **Preparation**
    - General anaesthesia (avoid drugs which may precipitate convulsions like ketamine)
    - Lateral recumbency (90° angle of the head, spine near the edge of the table)
    - Clip fur/disinfect skin

- **Technique**

Cisternal fluid puncture
    - Anatomical landmarks: occipital protuberance and wing of the atlas
    - Puncture site:
        Method 1: in the centre of a triangle between the occipital protuberance and the wing of the atlas (mild skin indentation)
        Method 2: in the middle of a line between the occipital protuberance and connecting line of both wings of the atlas (mild skin indentation)
    - Puncture:
        Method 1: advance the spinal needle containing a stylet (22 G) in a vertical manner, until the resistance of the dura mater (possibly including some skin twitches) has been overcome, remove the stylet
        Method 2: advance the spinal needle containing a stylet until the dura mater can be felt (slight resistance), remove the stylet, puncture the dura mater until the fluid flows freely
    - Obtaining the fluid: wait for it to drip passively into a sterile Eppendorf tube (0.5–1.0ml)
    - Ensure a calm post anaesthetic recovery

Lumbar fluid puncture
    - Anatomical land marks: spinous process L6 and iliac wing
    - Puncture site: cranial of the spinous process L6 (dog)/L7 (cat)
    - Puncture: advance the spinal needle containing a stylet (22 G) in a vertical to cranial direction and overcome the resistance of the dura mater. Push the needle forwards along the base of the spinal canal and pull the spinal needle back a little into the ventral subarachnoid space
    - Remove the stylet

- Obtaining the fluid: wait for it to drip passively into a sterile Eppendorf tube (0.5–1.0ml)
- Ensure a calm post-anaesthetic recovery

Complications

- Haemorrhage
- Convulsions
- Injury of the spinal cord
- Infection
- Respiratory arrest
- Brain herniation (in case of increased intracranial pressure)

Further Neurological Examination Methods

- Laboratory investigations
- Muscle biopsy
- Nerve biopsy
- Ultrasound examination (puppies with an open fontanel)
- Magnetic resonance imaging (MRI)
- Scintigraphy
- Epidurography
- Discography
- Electroencephalography (EEG)
- Electromyelography (EMG)
- Angiography

11 Ophthalmological Examination Methods

Case History

Principal Symptoms

- Loss of eyesight/blindness
- Red eye
- Ocular discharge
- Blepharospasm
- Exophthalmus/enophthalmus
- Strabismus
- Anisocoria

- Mydriasis/miosis
- Nystagmus
- Prolapse of the nictitating membrane
- Corneal/lens opacity
- Entropium/ectropium

Inspection

Indication

- Part of the opthalmological examination

Inspection

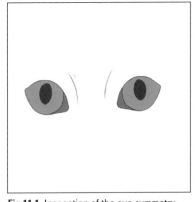

Fig 11.1 Inspection of the eye symmetry

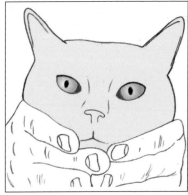

Fig 11.2 Inspection of the facial symmetry

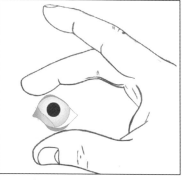

Fig 11.3 Inspection of the eye/conjunctivae

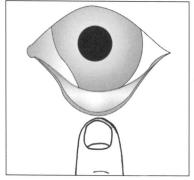

Fig 11.4 Inspection of the conjunctivae

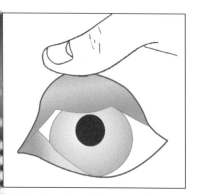

Fig 11.5 Inspection of the conjunctivae

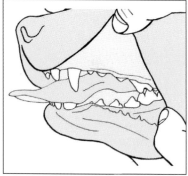

Fig 11.6 Inspection of the excretory ducts of the salivary glands

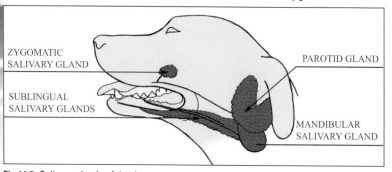

Fig 11.7 Salivary glands of the dog

Method

- **Technique**
  - Observe and examine the eyes/conjunctivae, face and oral cavity

Findings

- **Physiological**
  - Nothing abnormal to detect (NAD)

- **Pathological**

  Eyeball/globe
  - Nystagmus
  - Strabismus
  - Enophthalmus/exophthalmus
  - Microphthalmia

  Eyelids
  - Blepharospasm
  - Entropium/ectropium
  - Tumour/meibomian cyst/stye/dermoid
  - Trichiasis/dystichiasis/ectopic lashes
  - Atresia of the lacrimal duct opening
  - Blepharitis
  - Dental fistula

  Conjunctivae
  - Ocular discharge
  - Conjunctivitis/keratoconjunctivitis
  - Haematoma
  - Dermoid
  - Hyperplasia/prolapse of the nictitating gland (cherry eye)
  - Eversion of the cartilage of the nictitating membrane
  - Prolapse of the nictitating membrane

  Cornea
  - Keratitis/ulcus
  - Corneal opacity
  - Foreign body

  Pupils
  - Anisocoria (Horner syndrome: miosis, ptosis, enophthalmus)
  - Miosis/mydriasis

  Anterior eye chamber
  - Hyphaema/hypopyon

  Lens
  - Lens luxation
  - Lens opacity/cataract

Sight Test

Indication

- Part of the ophthalmological examination

Sight Test

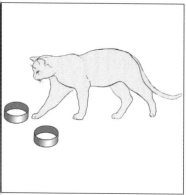

Fig 11.8 Obstacle course

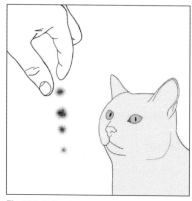

Fig 11.9 Following movement test

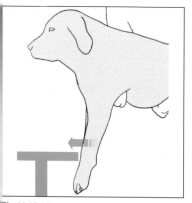

Fig 11.10 Visual placing response/table-edge test

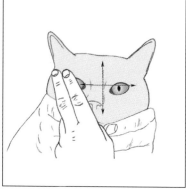

Fig 11.11 Eye mobility and movement

Method

- **Technique**

    Obstacle course
    - Observe the patient and his movements while negotiating an obstacle course and offering differing lighting conditions

    Following movement test
    - Observe the eye movements after dropping some cotton wool within the field of vision
    - Visual placing response/table-edge test

    Approach a table edge with the patient's forelimbs
    - Eye mobility and movement
    - Observe the eye movements when the patient is following the examiner's finger

Findings

- **Physiological**
    - Nothing abnormal to detect (NAD)

- **Pathological**
    - Partial loss of vision (uni-/bilateral)
    - Complete loss of vision/blindness (uni-/bilateral)

Reflexes

Indication

- Part of the general ophthalmological examination
- Suspected neurological disease

Reflexes

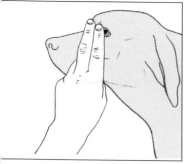

Fig 11.12 Menace response

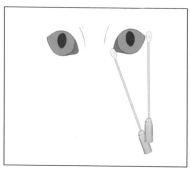

Fig 11.13 Palpebral reflex (blink reflex)

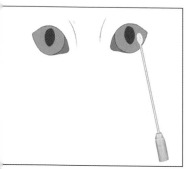

Fig 11.14 Corneal reflex

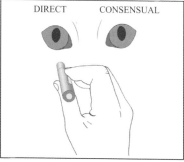

Fig 11.15 Pupillary light reflex (direct and consensual)

Method

- **Technique**

  Menace response
  - Quick movement with a finger towards the eye

  Palpebral reflex (blink reflex)
  - Touch the eyelids with a cotton bud

  Corneal reflex
  - Touch the cornea with a cotton bud

  Pupillary light reflex (PLR)
  - Direct: pupillary reaction of the lit eye
  - Consensual: pupillary reaction of the non-lit eye
  - Swinging flashlight test: make swinging movements with the light source from one eye to the other

Findings

- **Physiological**

  Menace response/palpebral reflex/corneal reflex
  - Blink

  Pupillary light reflex (PLR)
  - Direct: miosis
  - Consensual: miosis
  - Swinging flashlight test: miosis of the latterly lit eye

- **Pathological**

  Menace response
  - Absence (cranial nerve II, VII)

  Palpebral reflex
  - absence (cranial nerve V, VII)

  Corneal reflex
  - Absence (cranial nerve V, VII)

  Pupillary light reflex (PLR)
  - Direct: absence (lesion of the afferent and/or efferent nerves in the stimulated eye)
  - Consensual: absence (lesion of the afferent nerves in the stimulated eye and/or the efferent nerves in the contralateral eye)
  - Swinging flashlight test: the latterly lit eye is dilated (lesion of the afferent nerve in the latterly lit eye)

Penlight Examination

Indication

- Ophthalmoscopic pre-examination (without mydriasis)

Penlight Examination

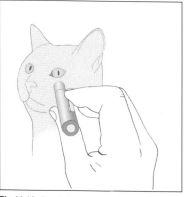

Fig 11.16 Penlight is shone directly into the eye

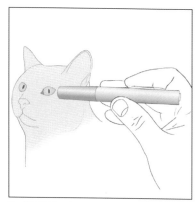

Fig 11.17 Penlight is shone from lateral through the anterior chamber

Method

- **Technique**
  - Shining the pen light into the eye from the front and lateral

Schirmer Tear Test

Indication

- Part of the ophthalmological examination
- Dry conjunctivae

Schirmer Tear Test

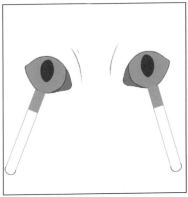

Fig 11.18 Schirmer Test Strip

Method

- **Technique**
  - Insert the Schirmer test strips into the lower lateral conjunctiva, place the notch at the edge of the lid
  - Hold both eyelids shut
  - Take the reading of the tear production after 1 min

Findings

- **Physiological**
  - Normal values: dog (21.9 ± 4.0 mm), cat (20.2 ± 4.5 mm)

- **Pathological**
  - Absence (cranial nerve VII, keratoconjunctivitis sicca)

Taking a Swab Sample

Indication

- Keratoconjunctivitis

Taking a Swab Sample

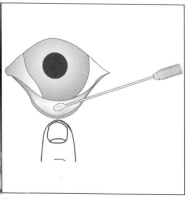

Fig 11.19 Taking a swab sample of the lower conjunctiva

Method

- **Technique**
  - Take a conjunctival swab with a cotton swab
  - Transfer it into a culture medium

Fluorescein Test

Indication

- Corneal injury/ulcer
- Patency test of the nasolacrimal duct

Fluorescein Test

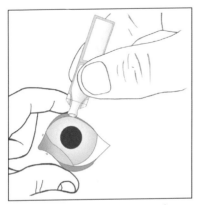

Fig 11.20 Administration of fluorescein

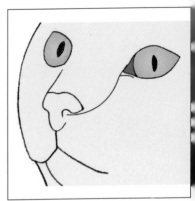

Fig 11.21 Course of the nasolacrimal duct

Method

- **Technique**
  - Administer fluorescein/Rose of Bengal drops into the eye

Findings

- **Physiological**
  - Nothing abnormal to detect (NAD)
  - Staining of the nostril

- **Pathological**
  - Staining of the cornea: epithelial defect
  - No staining of the nostril: nasolacrimal duct stenosis

Eversion of the Nictitating Membrane

Indication

- Part of the ophthalmological examination

Eversion of the Nictitating Membrane

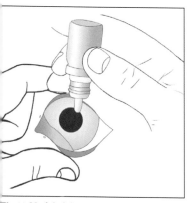

Fig 11.22 Administration of topical anaesthesia

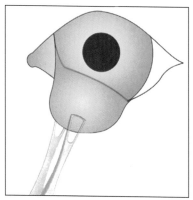

Fig 11.23 Eversion of the nictitating membrane

Method

- **Technique**
  - Administer 1–2 drops of topical anaesthesia suitable for the eye (oxybuprocaine 0.4 per cent)
  - Evert the nictitating membrane with an atraumatic pair of tweezers

Findings

- **Physiological**
  - Nothing abnormal to detect (NAD)

- **Pathological**
  - Prolapse of the nictitating gland
  - Eversion of the cartilage of the nictitating membrane
  - Foreign body
  - Follicular conjunctivitis

Gonioscopy

Indication

- Evaluation of the iridocorneal angle in case of glaucoma

Gonioscopy

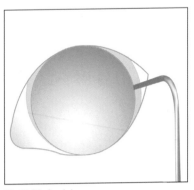

Fig 11.24 Goniolens

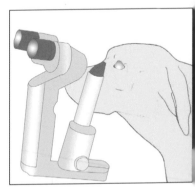

Fig 11.25 Slit lamp examination

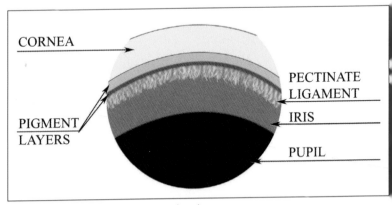

Fig 11.26 Morphology of the iridocorneal angle

Method

- **Preparation**
    - Administer 1–2 drops of topical anaesthesia suitable for the eye (oxybuprocaine 0.4 per cent)

- **Technique**
    - Place the contact lens onto the cornea with the concave side facing the cornea
    - Administer physiological saline via a silicone hose
    - Apply slight pressure to the contact lens
    - Remove the syringe
    - Examine the iridocorneal angle from lateral with the slit lamp
    - Lift the silicone hose and release the contact lens

Findings

- **Physiological**
    - Presence of all physiological structures

- **Pathological**
    - Loss of a pigment band (angle closure glaucoma)

Tonometry

Indication

- Measure of the ocular pressure in cases of suspected glaucoma

Tonometry

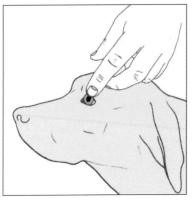

Fig 11.27 Comparative digital tonometry

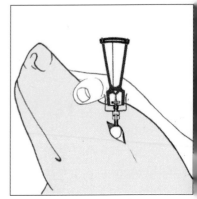

Fig 11.28 Tonometry with a Schiötz tonometer

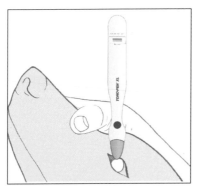

Fig 11.29 Tonometry with Tonopen®

Method

- **Preparation**
  - Topical anaesthesia
  - Patient sitting, possible dorsal or lateral recumbency

- **Technique**

  Schiötz tonometer
  - Attach 7.5g weight
  - Hold the eyelids open
  - Place the tonometer vertically and centrally onto the cornea
  - Record the scale reading
  - Repeat the procedure

  Tonopen®
  - Hold the eyelids open
  - Place the Tonopen vertically and centrally onto the cornea
  - Read the measure in mm Hg
  - Repeat the procedure

Findings

- **Physiological**

  Schiötz tonometer
  - Normal values: 9.5 (c. 15mm Hg)–5.5 (c. 30mm Hg)

  Tonopen®
  - Normal values: 15–30mm Hg

- **Pathological**

  Schiötz tonometer
  - < 5.5 (> 30mm Hg) (glaucoma)

  Tonopen®
  - > 30mm Hg (glaucoma)

Flushing of the Nasolacrimal Duct

Indication

- Testing the patency of the nasolacrimal duct

Flushing of the Nasolacrimal Duct

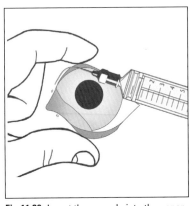

Fig 11.30 Insert the cannula into the upper lacrimal duct opening

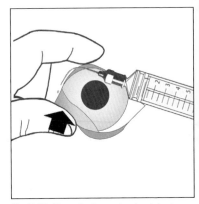

Fig 11.31 Keep the lower lacrimal duct opening shut and flush

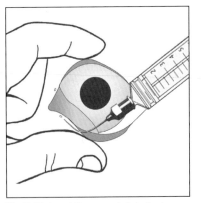

Fig 11.32 Insert the cannula into the lower lacrimal duct opening

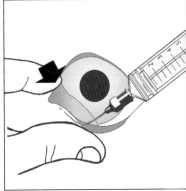

Fig 11.33 Keep the upper lacrimal duct shut and flush

Examination During Pupillary Dilation: Ophthalmoscopy

Indication

- Part of the ocular examination (ocular fundus examination)

Ophthalmoscopy

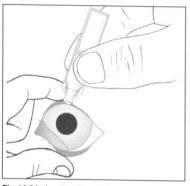

Fig 11.34 Application of the mydriatic eye drops

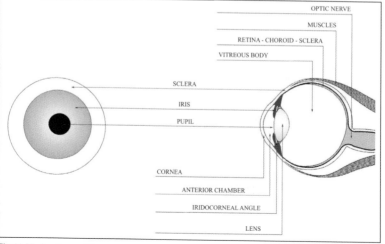

OPTIC NERVE

MUSCLES

RETINA - CHOROID - SCLERA

VITREOUS BODY

SCLERA

IRIS

PUPIL

CORNEA

ANTERIOR CHAMBER

IRIDOCORNEAL ANGLE

LENS

Fig 11.35 Anatomy of the eye

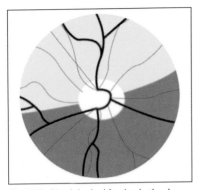

Fig 11.36 Physiological fundus in the dog

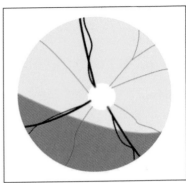

Fig 11.37 Physiological fundus in the cat

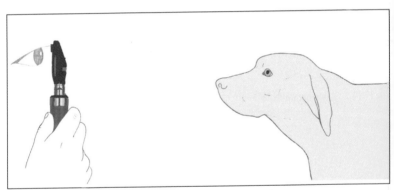

Fig 11.38 Direct ophthalmoscopy (examination from a distance)

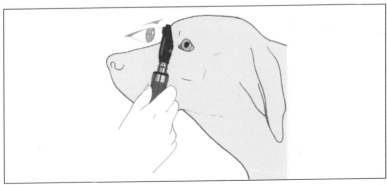

Fig 11.39 Direct ophthalmoscopy (close up examination)

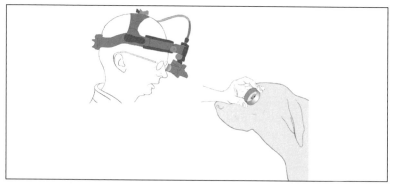

Fig 11.40 Indirect ophthalmoscopy (binocular headband ophthalmoscope)

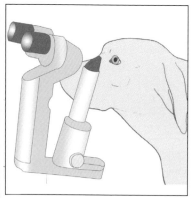

Fig 11.41 Slit lamp biomicroscopy

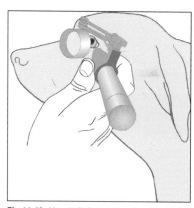

Fig 11.42 Hand slit lamp examination

Method

- **Preparation**
  - Mydriasis: tropicamide 1 per cent eye drops (mydriasis after c. 15 min) (antagonist: pilocarpine)
  - Darkened examination room

- **Technique**

  Direct ophthalmoscopy
  - Upright unreversed fundal image
  - Narrow visual field (c. 9°)
  - High magnification (c. 20 X)
    1. Set the lens to 0 dioptre
    2. Examine the eye from a distance: localise the red reflex c. 30cm away from the patient's eye, hold the ohthalmoscope closely to the examiner's eye, hold both eyes open, the examiner's right eye should examine the patient's right eye
    3. Examine the eye from close up: about 1–2cm away from the patient's eye, set the lens

  Indirect ophthalmoscopy
  - Upside down and reversed fundal image
  - Large visual field (c. 35°)
  - Low magnification (c. 4 X)
    1. Hold the lens about 2–3cm away from the patient's eye
    2. Examine the eye with a binocular headband ophthalmoscope about 30cm away from the patient's eye

  Hand slit lamp biomicroscopy
  - Variable beam width suitable for localisation and classification of cataracts

Findings

- **Physiological**
  - Nothing abnormal to detect (NAD)

- **Pathological**

  Cornea
  - Keratitis
  - Ulcus
  - Oedema
  - Foreign body
  - Dermoid
  - Keratoconjunctivitis sicca
  - Lipid dystrophy

  Anterior chamber
  - Uveitis anterior
  - Hyphaema
  - Hypopyon
  - Iritis/iridocyclitis
  - Iridal coloboma/cyst
  - Iris bombé
  - Synechiae
  - Tumour (melanoma/ciliary body adenoma/adenocarcinoma)
  - Foreign body

  Lens
  - Lens luxation
  - Cataract

  Posterior chamber/vitreous body
  - Uveitis posterior
  - Fundal haemorrhage
  - Foreign body

  Ocular fundus
  - Retinal atrophy (progressive retinal atrophy/PRA)
  - Retinal detachment
  - Collie eye anomaly (CEA)
  - Coloboma
  - Chorioretinitis
  - Neuritis of the optical nerve/papillary oedema
  - Hypoplasia of the optical nerve

X-Ray Study

Indication

- Suspected tumour or foreign body

X-Ray Study

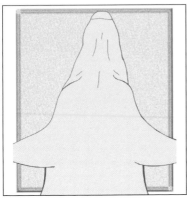

Fig 11.43 Head (dorsoventral view)   **Fig 11.44** Head (lateral view)

Method

- **Technique**
  - Head (dorsoventral and lateral view)

Findings

- **Physiological**
  - Nothing abnormal to detect (NAD)

- **Pathological**
  - Tumour (± osteolysis)
  - Foreign body

Ultrasound Examination

Indication

- Suspected tumour, lens luxation, haemorrhage, retinal detachment, foreign body, retrobulbar process

Ultrasound Examination

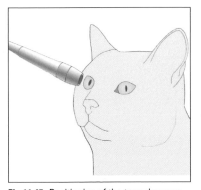

Fig 11.45 Positioning of the transducer on the cornea

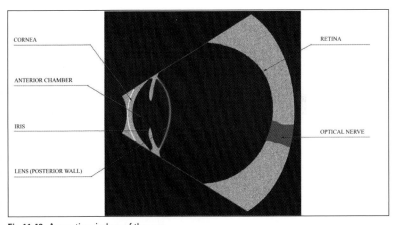

CORNEA

ANTERIOR CHAMBER

IRIS

LENS (POSTERIOR WALL)

RETINA

OPTICAL NERVE

Fig 11.46 Acoustic window of the eye

Method

- **Preparation**
  - B-Mode
  - Eye socket: 5–7.5 MHz transducer
  - Eyeball: 10–12.5 MHz transducer
  - Stand-off pad
  - Topical anaesthesia topicamide 1 per cent

- **Technique**
  - Apply the ultrasound gel to the transducer
  - Position the transducer directly onto the cornea or alternatively onto the closed eyelids

Findings

- **Physiological**
  - Nothing abnormal to detect (NAD)

- **Pathological**
  - Lens luxation
  - Cataract
  - Tumour
  - Hyphaema/hypopyon
  - Granuloma
  - Parasites
  - Retinal detachment
  - Foreign body
  - Retrobulbar abscess/tumour/mucocele

Biopsy

Indication

• Tissue sampling for histological/cytological examination

Biopsy

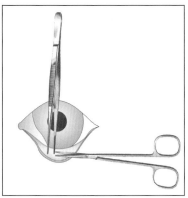

Fig 11.47 Biopsy of the conjunctiva

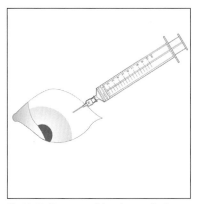

Fig 11.48 Puncture of the vitreous body

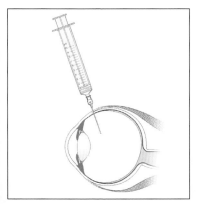

Fig 11.49 Puncture of the vitreous body

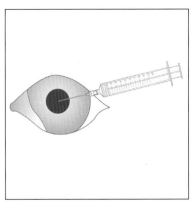 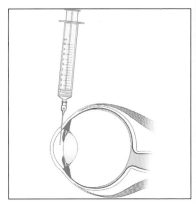

Figs 11.50 and 11.51 Puncture of the anterior chamber

Method

- **Preparation**

    Puncture
    – Sedation/general anaesthesia
    – Puncture needle: 25 G

    Biopsy of the conjunctiva
    – Topical anaesthesia: topicamide 1 per cent

- **Technique**

    Puncture of the vitreous body
    – Puncture site: lateral canthus towards the middle of the eyeball
    – Aspirate c. 0.2–0.3ml

    Puncture of the anterior chamber
    – Puncture site: lateral pupillary border towards iris
    – Aspirate c. 0.2–0.3ml

    Biopsy of the conjunctiva
    – Elevate a mucosal fold with a pair of forceps
    – Make a skin incision with a pair of scissors
    – Leave the wound open

Further Ophthalmological Examination Methods

- Laboratory investigations
- Electroretinography (ERG)
- Computed tomography (CT)
- Magnetic resonance tomography (MRT)
- Biopsy (retrobulbar, conjunctiva, anterior chamber, vitreous body, muscle)
- Fluorescence angiography
- Sialography
- Dacryocysteography
- Optical coherence tomography (OCT)
- Visually evoked cortical potentials (VECP)
- Confocal laser scanning tomography (CLST)

12 Otological Examination Methods

Case History

Principal Symptoms

- Head shaking/scratching
- Head tilt
- Nystagmus
- Ataxia

Inspection

Indication

- Part of the general examination

Inspection

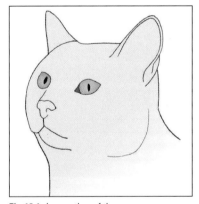

Fig 12.1 Inspection of the ear position/posture

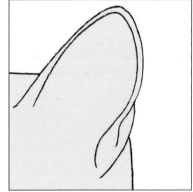

Fig 12.2 Inspection of the pinna

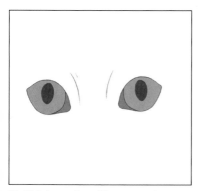

Fig 12.3 Inspection of the eyes and eye movements

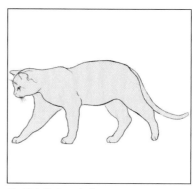

Fig 12.4 Gait analysis

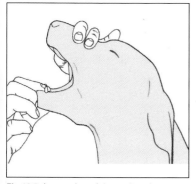

Fig 12.5 Inspection of the oral cavity

Method

- **Technique**
  - Observation of the head and ear position, gait, external ear, eyes and oral cavity

Findings

- **Physiological**
  - Nothing abnormal to detect (NAD)

- **Pathological**

  Head/ear position
  - Head tilt (damage on the same side)
  - Head-shaking

  External ear
  - Discharge from the ear
  - Tumour/polyp
  - Necrosis of the pinnal edge
  - Aural haematoma

  Eyes
  - Nystagmus

  Gait
  - Ataxia

  Oral cavity
  - Nasopharyngeal polyp

Olfactory Test

Indication

- Part of the aural examination

Olfactory Test

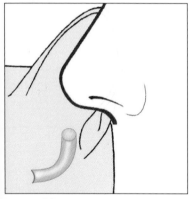

Fig 12.6 Olfactory test

Method

- **Technique**
  - Smell the external ear

Findings

- **Physiological**
  - Nothing abnormal to detect (NAD)

- **Pathological**
  - Purulent
  - Malassezia-like

Otoscopy

Indication

- Ear disease

Otoscopy

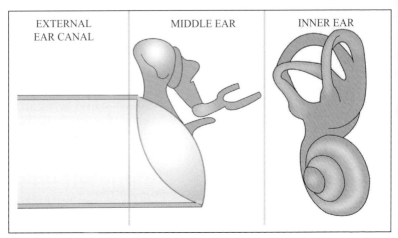

Fig 12.7 Anatomical regions of the ear

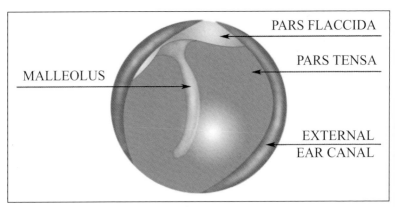

Fig 12.8 Tympanic membrane, otoscopic view

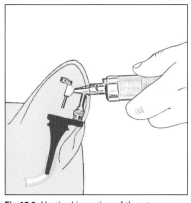

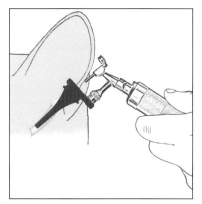

Fig 12.9 Vertical insertion of the otoscope funnel

Fig 12.10 Horizontal advancement of the otoscope funnel

Method

- **Technique**
  - Attach a suitable funnel to the otoscope
  - Insert the funnel vertically at first, then advance it horizontally while examining the external ear canal
  - Evaluate the tympanic membrane

Findings

- **Physiological**
  - Nothing abnormal to detect (NAD)

- **Pathological**
  - Otitis externa
  - Otitis media
  - Foreign body (grass seed/awn)
  - Tumour/polyp
  - Ruptured tympanic membrane

X-Ray Study

Indication

- Suspected otitis media

X-Ray Study

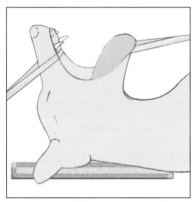

Fig 12.11 View of the tympanic bulla

Method

- **Technique**
  - Sedation
  - X-ray view through the open mouth

Findings

- **Physiological**
  - Nothing abnormal to detect (NAD)

- **Pathological**
  - Radiopacity of the tympanic bulla (otitis media, tumour)

Biopsy

Indication

- *Otitis externa* of unknown origin

Swab Sample

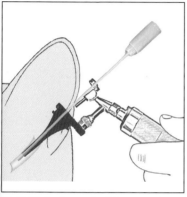

Fig 12.12 Swab sample of the external ear canal

Method

- **Technique**
  - Take a swab sample from the ear canal and/or the discharge while having visual control through the otoscope
  - Transfer the sample into a culture medium (bacterial/mycotic examinations)

Hearing Test

Indication

- Suspected hearing loss/deafness

Hearing Test

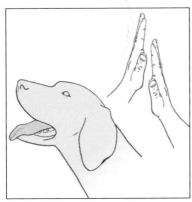

Fig 12.13 Subjective hearing test

Method

- **Technique**
  - Clap your hands, call and whistle as rough indicator for the patient's hearing ability

  Objective hearing tests
  - Audibly evoked potentials (AEP)
  - Brainstem auditory evoked response audiometry (BAERA)

Further Otological Examination Methods

- Laboratory investigations
- Audibly evoked potentials (AEP)
- Brain auditory evoked response audiometry (BAERA)
- Computed tomography (CT)
- Magnetic resonance tomography (MRT)

13 Dermatological Examination Methods

Case History

Principal Symptoms

- Pruritus
- Alopecia
- Efflorescences of the skin

Inspection

Indication

- Part of the general examination

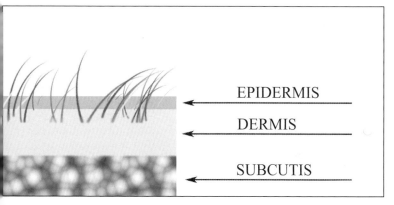

Fig 13.1 Anatomical structures of the skin

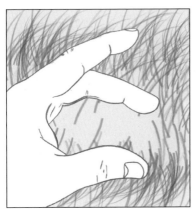

Fig 13.2
Inspection of the skin and hair

Method

- **Technique**
  - Inspect the hair, skin, mucocutaneous junctions and mucous membranes

- **Evaluation criteria**
  - Completeness of the coat, colour and symmetry

Classification of Skin Lesions: Primary Efflorescences

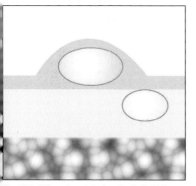

Fig 13.3 Blister/vesicle (vesicula/bulla)

Fig 13.4 Spot (macula)

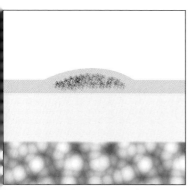

Fig 13.5 Nodule (papula/plaque)

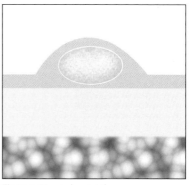

Fig 13.6 Pimple (pustula)

Fig 13.7 Wheal (urticaria)

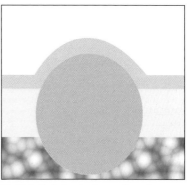

Fig 13.8 Node (nodus/tumour)

Classification of Skin Lesions: Secondary Efflorescences

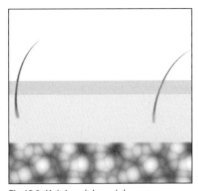

Fig 13.9 Hair loss (alopecia)

Fig 13.10 Atrophy

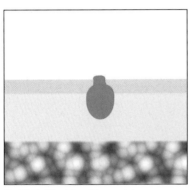

Fig 13.11 Black head (comedo)

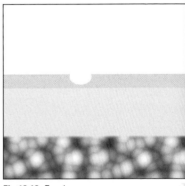

Fig 13.12 Erosion

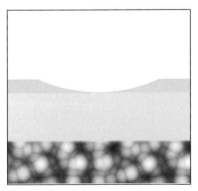

Fig 13.13 Excoriation

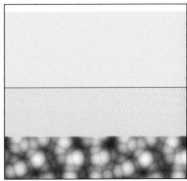

Fig 13.14 Hyperkeratosis

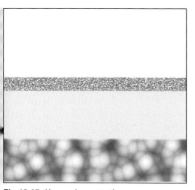

Fig 13.15 Hyperpigmentation

Fig 13.16 Hypopigmentation

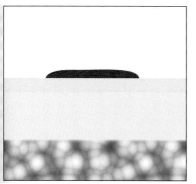

Fig 13.17 Crust (crusta)

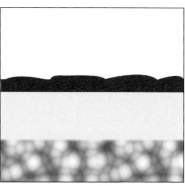

Fig 13.18 Eruption/lichenification

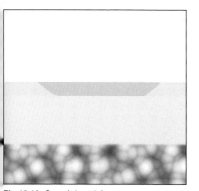

Fig 13.19 Scar (cicatrix)

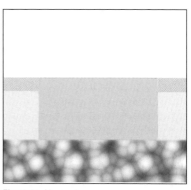

Fig 13.20 Necrosis

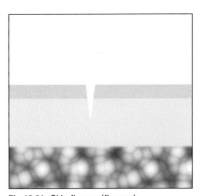

Fig 13.21 Skin fissure (fissura)

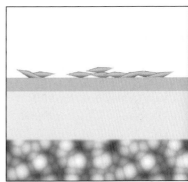

Fig 13.22 Scale (squama)

Fig 13.23 Ulcus

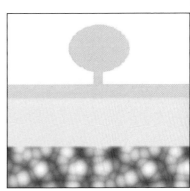

Fig 13.24 Wart/papilloma

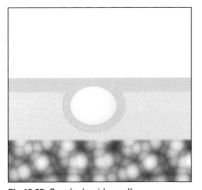

Fig 13.25 Cyst (subepidermal)

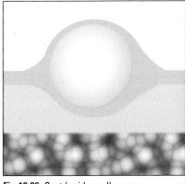

Fig 13.26 Cyst (epidermal)

Inspection: Distribution of Lesions

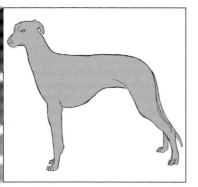

Fig 13.27 Generalised

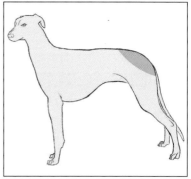

Fig 13.28 Localised

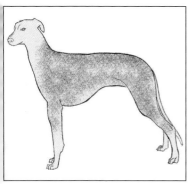

Fig 13.29 Disseminated

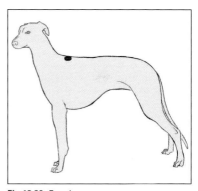

Fig 13.30 Focal

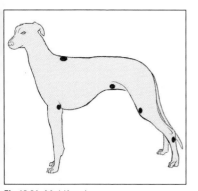

Fig 13.31 Multifocal

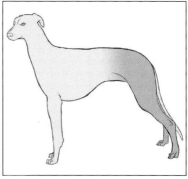

Fig 13.32 Regional

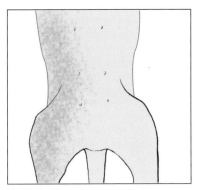

Fig 13.33 Bilateral asymmetrical

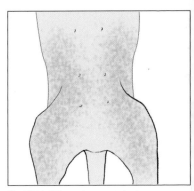

Fig 13.34 Bilateral symmetrical

Findings

- **Physiological**
  - Nothing abnormal to detect (NAD)

- **Pathological**

  Skin colour/colour of mucous membranes
  - Yellow: icterus
  - Blue: cyanosis
  - White: shock, anaemia
  - Red: hyperaemia, septicaemia, CO-poisoning, polycythaemia

  Primary efflorescences
  - Blister/vesicle (vesicula/bulla)
  - Spot (macula)
  - Node (nodus/tumour/tuber)
  - Nodule (papule)
  - Pimple (pustule)
  - Wheal (urticaria)

Secondary skin efflorescences
  - Hair loss (alopecia)
  - Atrophy
  - Black head (comedo)
  - Erosion
  - Ulcus
  - Excoriation
  - Hyperkeratosis
  - Hyper-/hypopigmentation
  - Crust (crusta)
  - Eruption/lichenification
  - Scar (cicatrix)
  - Necrosis
  - Skin fissure (fissura)
  - Scale (squama)
  - Wart/papilloma
  - Cyst

Distribution of skin lesions
  - Generalised
  - Localised
  - Focal/multifocal
  - Regional
  - Bilateral symmetrical/asymmetrical

Palpation

Indication

- Part of the dermatological examination

Palpation

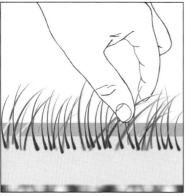

Fig 13.35 Palpation of the hair

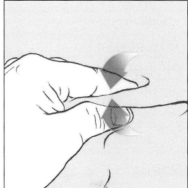

Fig 13.36 Palpation of the skin

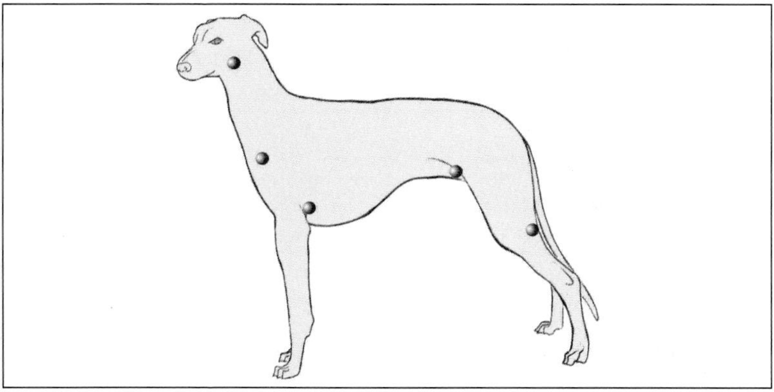

Fig 13.37 Location of lymph nodes (dogs)

Method

- **Technique**

  Hair
  - Palpate the hair and evaluate its firmness, dampness, structure and colour

  Skin
  - Palpate the epidermis by rolling the skin between your fingers
  - Palpate the subcutaneous tissues
  - Test the turgor: elevate the skin, then let go of it and measure the time that lapses until the skin fold has disappeared

  Lymph nodes
  - Undertake comparative palpation of the lymph nodes: parotid lymph nodes, mandibular lymph nodes, superficial cervical lymph nodes (prescapular lymph nodes), axillary lymph nodes, superficial inguinal lymph nodes, popliteal lymph nodes

Findings

- **Physiological**
  - Nothing abnormal to detect (NAD)

- **Pathological**

  Hair
  - Seborrhoea
  - Dry, brittle hair

  Skin
  - Calcinosis cutis
  - Tumour
  - Atheroma
  - Elbow callus (hygroma)
  - Cyst
  - Comedone
  - Wart/papilloma
  - Skin turgor: dehydration, Ehlers-Danlos syndrome

  Lymph nodes
  - Lymphadenopathy

Olfactory Test

Indication

- Part of the dermatological examination

Olfactory Test

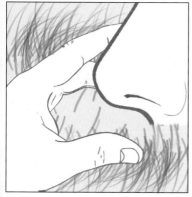

Fig 13.38 Olfactory test

Method

- **Technique**
  - Smell the skin

Findings

- **Physiological**
  - Nothing abnormal to detect (NAD)

- **Pathological**
  - Purulent
  - Malassezia-like

Flea Check with a Flea Comb

Indication

• Ectoparasites

Flea Check with Flea Comb

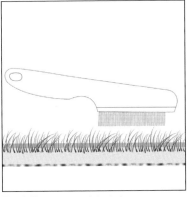

Fig 13.39 Combing of the hair

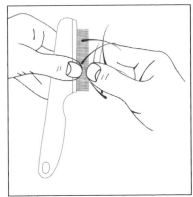

Fig 13.40 Examination of the sample material

Method

• **Technique**
  – Comb the hair with a flea comb, examine the combed material (macroscopically and microscopically)

Findings

• **Physiological**
  – Nothing abnormal to detect (NAD)

• **Pathological**
  – Ectoparasites
  – Fleas
  – Ticks
  – Mites
  – Lice
  – Biting lice

Wood-Lamp Examination

Indication

- Dermatophytes

Wood-Lamp Examination

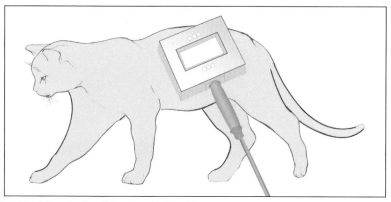

Fig 13.41 Examination of the skin with Wood-lamp

Method

- **Technique**
  - Darken the examination room
  - Illuminate the hair/skin with an ultraviolet light (Wood–lamp)
  - Evaluate the fluorescence

Findings

- **Physiological**
  - Absence of fluorescence

- **Pathological**
  - Fluorescence (*Microsporum* spp.)

Skin Scrape

Indication

- Cytological examination

Skin Scrape

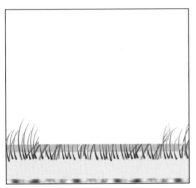

Fig 13.42 Clip the fur

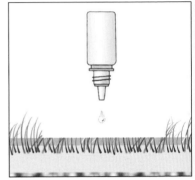

Fig 13.43 Application of paraffin oil

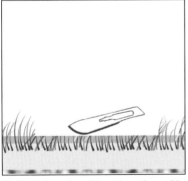

Fig 13.44 Scraping of the skin surface with a scalpel blade

Skin Scrape: Crushing Preparation

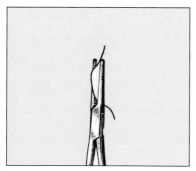

Fig 13.45 Crush a skin fold with a pair of Pean forceps

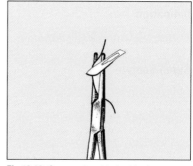

Fig 13.46 Scrape the skin inside the crushed skin fold

Method

- **Technique: skin scrape**
  - Clip the fur
  - Apply paraffin onto skin
  - Scrape the skin while holding the scalpel blade perpendicular to the direction of the fur (superficial scrape/deep scrape)
  - Transfer the sample to a microscope slide/cover slide for microscopic examination

  Crushing preparation
  - Clip the fur
  - Crush a skin fold with a Pean forceps
  - Apply paraffin oil to the skin
  - Scrape the skin with the scalpel blade perpendicular to the direction of the fur
  - Transfer the sample to a microscope slide/cover slide for microscopic examination

Findings

- **Physiological**
  - Nothing abnormal to detect (NAD)

- **Pathological**

  Ectoparasites
  - Mites (especially Demodex sp.)

  Fungi
  - Microsporum sp., Trichophyton sp.
  - Candida sp., Malassezia sp.

Swab Sample

Indication

- Bacterial/mycological examination

Swab Sample

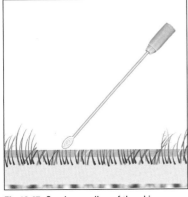

Fig 13.47 Swab sampling of the skin

Method

- **Technique**
  - Part and clip the fur
  - Take a swab of the skin with a cotton swab
  - Transfer the swab sample to a culture medium

Findings

- **Physiological**
  - Nothing abnormal to detect (NAD)

- **Pathological**
  - Bacteria
  - Fungi

Sticky Tape Impression Smear

Indication

- Dermatophytosis, ectoparasites

Sticky Tape Impression Smear

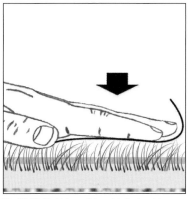

Fig 13.48 Dabbing of the skin/hair with sticky tape

Method

- **Technique**
  - Dab the skin or hair with a strip of sticky tape
  - Place the strip onto a microscope slide and examine the sample with the microscope

Findings

- **Physiological**
  - Nothing abnormal to detect (NAD)

- **Pathological**

  Ectoparasites
  - Fleas/flea dirt
  - Mites
  - Lice/nits
  - Biting lice

  Fungi
  - Microsporum sp., Trichophyton sp.
  - Candida sp., Malassezia sp.

Hair Pluck Sample

Indication

- Examination of the hair
- Fungal culture

Hair Sample

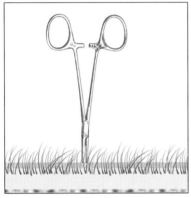

Fig 13.49 Hair sampling

Method

- **Technique**
  - Pluck some hair from around the edge of a skin lesion
  - Process the sample for an examination or a fungal culture

Findings

- **Physiological**
  - Nothing abnormal to detect (NAD)

- **Pathological**

  Examination of the hair
  - Hair root dystrophy
  - Hair breakage/brittleness
  - Hair growth phase (telogen/anagen phase)

  Fungi
  - Microsporum sp., Trichophyton sp.

Skin Punch Biopsy

Indication

• Histological examination

Skin Punch Biopsy

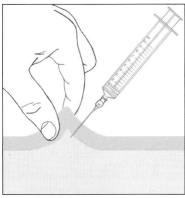

Fig 13.50 Topical anaesthesia

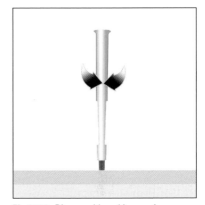

Fig 13.51 Biopsy with a skin punch

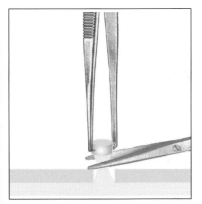

Fig 13.52 Removal of the sample

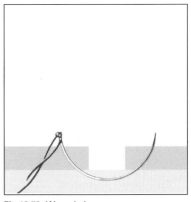

Fig 13.53 Wound closure

Fine Needle Biopsy

Indication

- Cytological examination of tumours

Fine Needle Biopsy

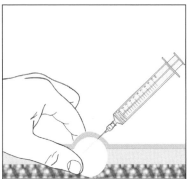

Fig 13.54 Fine needle aspiration

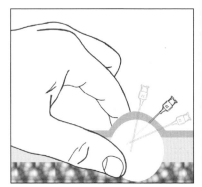

Fig 13.55 Fine needle punch technique

Method

- **Technique**

   Skin punch biopsy
   - Clip the fur
   - Disinfect the skin
   - Topical anaesthesia (lidocaine 1 per cent)
   - Make skin incision by creating rotating movements with the biopsy punch
   - Remove the sample and cut the subcutaneous tissue off
   - Transfer the sample into a fixation medium
   - Close the skin with sutures or staples

   Fine needle aspiration
   - Puncture the tumour with a hypodermic needle and attached syringe
   - Aspirate and remove the puncture needle
   - Transfer the sample onto a microscope slide for cytological examination

Fine needle punch technique
- Puncture the tumour with a hypodermic needle only (without a syringe)
- Pierce the tumour tissue multiple times
- Transfer the sample onto a microscope slide by using an air filled syringe and examine cytologically

Findings

- **Physiological**
  - Nothing abnormal to detect (NAD)

- **Pathological**
  - Inflammation
  - Tumour

Further Dermatological Examination Methods

- **Laboratory investigations**
  - Blood analysis
  - Pathogen serology (Sarcoptes sp.)
  - Monoclonal allergy tests
  - Endocrine function tests
  - Urinary analysis
  - Faecal analysis

- **Allergy test**

Part II
Treatment Methods

14 Injection

Subcutaneous Injection

Indication

- Injection of injection solutions
- Injection of vaccinations

Subcutaneous Injection

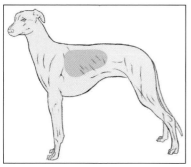

Fig 14.1 Subcutaneous injection areas

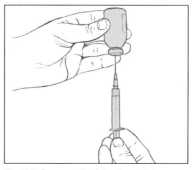

Fig 14.2 Draw up the injection solution

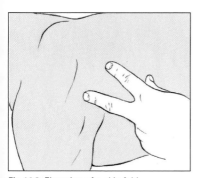

Fig 14.3 Elevation of a skin fold

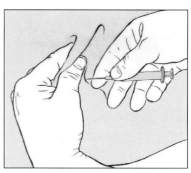

Fig 14.4 Skin puncture and injection

Method

- **Technique**
  - Injection needle (20–22 G)
  - Disinfect the puncture membrane with an alcohol swab
  - Draw up the injection solution without introducing air into the bottle and remove any air from the syringe
  - Elevate a skin fold with three fingers
  - Puncture the skin tangentially below the thumb of the left hand
  - Perform the puncture against the hair line (from caudal to cranial)
  - Injection needle must be freely mobile to either side
  - Inject
  - Remove the injection needle

  Injection areas
  - Lateral thoracic wall

Complications

- Extracutaneous malinjection (penetration of two layers of skin)
- Injuries to muscles, bones and cutaneous nerve tissue
- Thorax puncture
- Abscess
- Necrosis

Intramuscular Injection

Indication

- Injection of injection solutions

Intramuscular injection in the dog

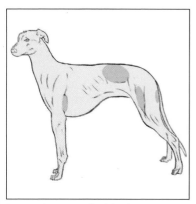

Fig 14.5 Intramuscular injection areas

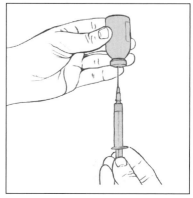

Fig 14.6 Draw up the injection solution into the syringe

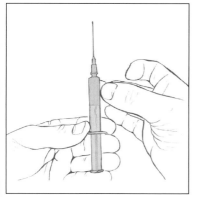

Fig 14.7 Removal of air bubbles from the syringe

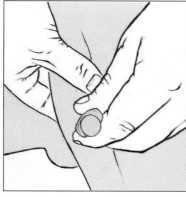

Fig 14.8 Quadriceps muscle of the thigh

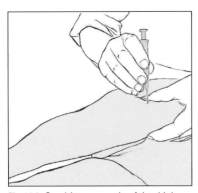

Fig 14.9 Quadriceps muscle of the thigh (cranial view)

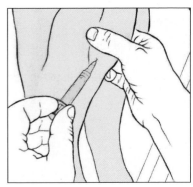

Fig 14.10 Semitendinous muscle/ semimembranous muscle

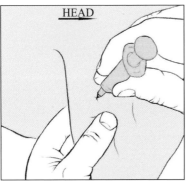

Fig 14.11 Triceps muscle of the forelimb

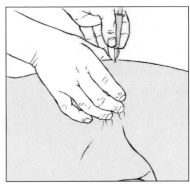

Fig 14.12 Dorsal lumbar musculature

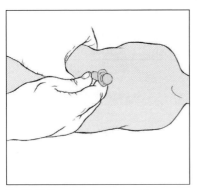

Fig 14.13 Dorsal lumbar musculature

Intramuscular Injection in the Cat

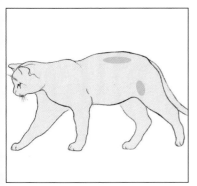

Fig 14.14 Intramuscular injection areas

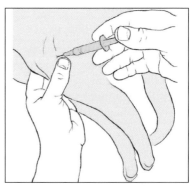

Fig 14.15 Quadriceps muscle of the thigh (fixation from cranial)

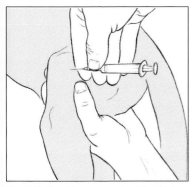

Fig 14.16 Quadriceps muscle of the thigh (fixation from caudal)

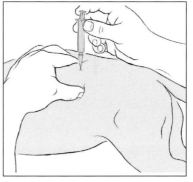

Fig 14.17 Dorsal lumbar musculature

Method

- **Preparation**

  Injection areas in the dog
  - Quadriceps muscle of the thigh
  - Semitendinous muscle/semimembranous muscle, take care with the sciatic nerve!
  - Triceps muscle of the forelimb
  - Dorsal lumbar musculature

  Injection areas in the cat
  - Quadriceps muscle of the thigh
  - Dorsal lumbar musculature

- **Technique**
  - Injection needle (thin lumen 24–25 G)
  - Disinfect the puncture membrane with an alcohol swab
  - Draw up the injection solution without introducing air into the bottle
  - Remove any air bubbles from the syringe
  - Fixate the muscle
  - Disinfect the skin with an alcohol swab
  - Tap the injection site and quickly puncture the muscle
  - Aspirate
  - Inject slowly
  - Remove the injection needle quickly

Complications

- Painfulness
- Aspiration of blood
- Paralysis/lesions of the sciatic nerve
- Abscess
- Muscle necrosis
- Intraarterial injection
- Anaphylactic shock

Intravenous Injection

Indication

- Injection of injection solutions

Intravenous Injection

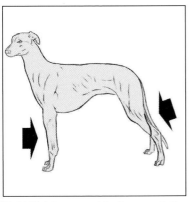

Fig 14.18 Intravenous injection areas in the dog

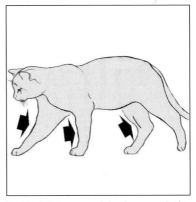

Fig 14.19 Intravenous injection areas in the cat

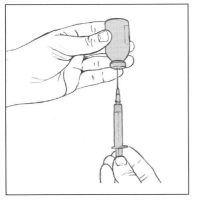

Fig 14.20 Injection solution is drawn up airfree

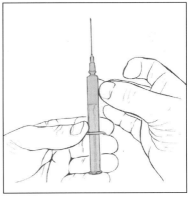

Fig 14.21 Air bubbles are removed from the syringe

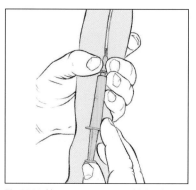

Fig 14.22 Venous puncture and injection

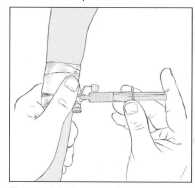

Fig 14.23 Injection with an intravenous butterfly catheter

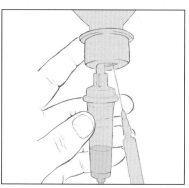

Fig 14.24 Injection by adding medication to an infusion bottle

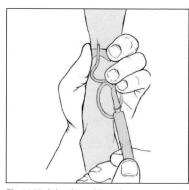

Fig 14.25 Injection via an intravenous catheter (injection port)

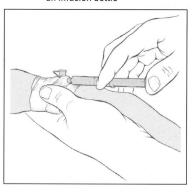

Fig 14.26 Injection via an intravenous catheter (infusion port)

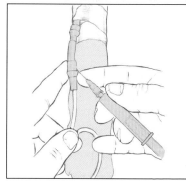

Fig 14.27 Injection via an infusion line

Method

- **Preparation**
  - Hypodermic needle (20–22 G) and syringe
  - Disinfect the puncture membrane with an alcohol swab
  - Draw up the injection solution without introducing any air into the bottle
  - Remove any air bubbles from the syringe

Venous puncture sites in the dog
  - Cephalic vein of the forelimb, lateral saphenous vein

Venous puncture sites in the cat
  - Cephalic vein of the forelimb, medial saphenous vein

- **Technique**

Venous puncture
  - Raise the vein
  - Perform a venous puncture with a hypodermic needle or a butterfly catheter
  - Attach a syringe once the blood flow is confirmed
  - Release the raised vein
  - Inject slowly
  - Remove the puncture needle or catheter while compressing the puncture site with swabs
  - Apply a small dressing

Injection via injection port
  - Remove the hypodermic needle from the syringe
  - Attach the syringe to the injection port of the intravenous catheter
  - Inject slowly

Injection via infusion port
  - Remove the hypodermic needle from the syringe
  - Remove the mandrel from the venous catheter
  - Attach the syringe to the infusion port of the intravenous catheter
  - Inject slowly

Injection via infusion line
  - Block the infusion line by bending or pinching it
  - Puncture the rubber membrane on the infusion line with the injection needle
  - Open the infusion line
  - Inject slowly

Complications

- Paravenous injection
- Thrombophlebitis
- Necrosis
- Anaphylaxis/shock

Intraperitoneal Injection

Indication

- Euthanasia

Intraperitoneal Injection

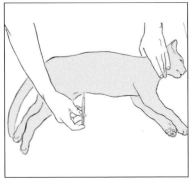

Fig 14.28 Intraperitoneal injection in lateral recumbency

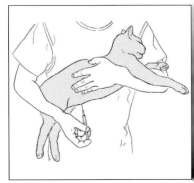

Fig 14.29 Intraperitoneal injection while holding the cat on your arm

Method

- **Technique**
  - Hypodermic needle (22–24 G) and syringe
  - Draw up the injection solution
  - Remove any air bubbles from the syringe
  - Change the hypodermic needle (especially with barbiturates)
  - Tap the injection site slightly (periumbilical/median)
  - Puncture the abdominal cavity while the syringe is attached
  - Check that the needle is freely mobile inside the abdominal cavity
  - Inject slowly
  - Remove the needle and syringe
  - Compress the puncture site digitally for about 1 min

Complications

- Inefficacy of the drug used
- Painfulness if accidental subcutaneous injection

Intracardiac Injection

Indication

- Reanimation
- Last resort in choice of euthanasia during deep general anaesthesia

Intracardiac Injection

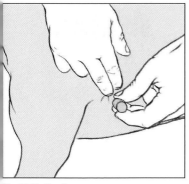

Fig 14.30 Cardiac puncture

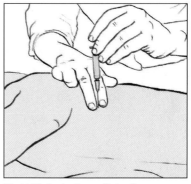

Fig 14.31 Aspiration and injection

Method

- **Technique**
  - Hypodermic needle (20–22 G) and syringe
  - Draw up the injection solution
  - Remove any air bubbles from the syringe
  - In case of euthanasia: deep general anaesthesia
  - Patient positioning (preferably in left lateral recumbency
  - Puncture site fourth–fifth intercostal space near the costochondral junction (cranial edge of the rib)
  - Perform the puncture in a vertical manner while aspirating permanently until the blood is aspirated in gushes
  - Inject
  - Remove the needle quickly in the insertion angle

Complications

- Atrial fibrillation
- Haemorrhages (haemothorax/haemoperi-cardium)
- Pneumothorax/perforation of the lung
- Infection

Intraarticular Injection

Indication

- Injection of injection solutions

Intraarticular Injection

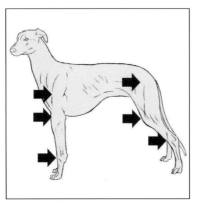

Fig 14.32 Intraarticular injection sites in the dog

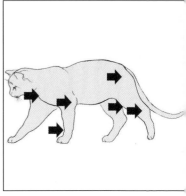

Fig 14.33 Intraarticular injection sites in the cat

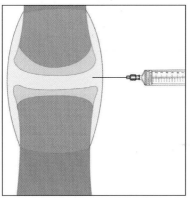

Fig 14.34 Puncture of the joint capsule

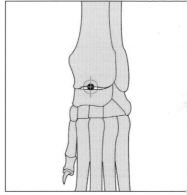

Fig 14.35 Carpal joint

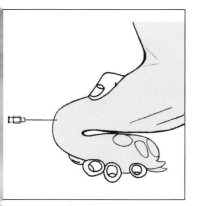

Fig 14.36 Flexed carpal joint

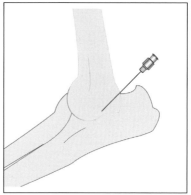

Fig 14.37 Elbow joint

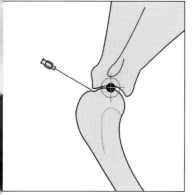

Fig 14.38 Shoulder joint

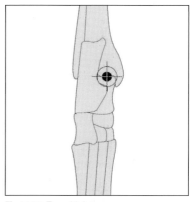

Fig 14.39 Tarsal joint

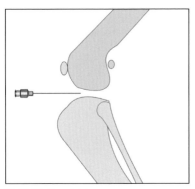

Fig 14.40 Knee joint

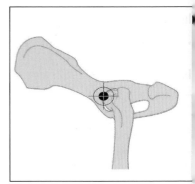

Fig 14.41 Hip joint

Method

- **Preparation**
  - Sedation
  - Partially flex the joints
  - Clip and disinfect the fur

- **Technique**
  - Palpate the joint effusion
  - Puncture the joint with a hypodermic needle (22 G) and an attached syringe
  - Aspirate synovia
  - Inject
  - Remove the hypodermic needle
  - Compress the puncture site

Complications

- Infection
- Haemorrhage
- Arthrosis as a result of cartilage injury

Injection at the Bicipital Tendon

Indication

- Therapeutic injection in case of tendovaginitis of the bicipital tendon

Injection at the Bicipital Tendon

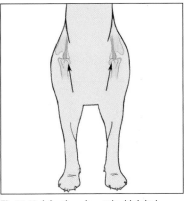

Fig 14.42 Injection site at the bicipital tendon

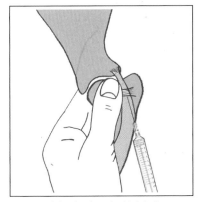

Fig 14.43 Injection into the bicipital groove

Method

- **Preparation**
  - Clip and disinfect the fur over the puncture site
  - Partially extend the upper limb

- **Technique**
  - Palpate the greater and minor tuberosity of the humerus
  - Puncture the skin with a hypodermic needle (22 G) and an attached syringe, slowly advance the needle into the bicipital groove
  - Inject one bolus, inject a second bolus while removing the needle
  - Remove the needle and syringe

Complications

- Joint puncture
- Bone puncture
- Puncture of the bicipital tendon
- Infection

Eye injection: Subconjunctival Injection

Indication

- Infection
- Allergy

Subconjunctival Injection

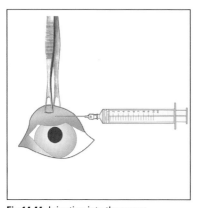

Fig 14.44 Injection into the upper conjunctiva

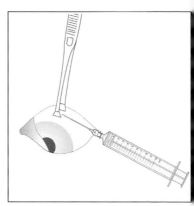

Fig 14.45 Injection into the conjunctiva

Method

- **Preparation**
  - Possibly light sedation

- **Technique**
  - Part the eyelids
  - Elevate the conjunctiva with an atraumatic pair of forceps
  - Puncture the conjunctiva in a tangential manner from lateral with a hypodermic needle and an attached syringe
  - Inject
  - Remove the needle and syringe

Complications

- Infection
- Puncture of the vitreous body

Eye injection: Injection into the Chamber of the Eye

Indication

- Infection
- Ocular haemorrhage (hyphaema)

Injection into the Chamber of the Eye

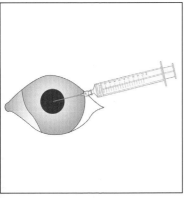

Fig 14.46 Injection into the anterior chamber

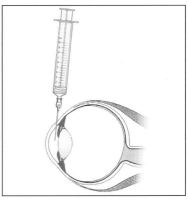

Fig 14.47 Injection into the anterior chamber

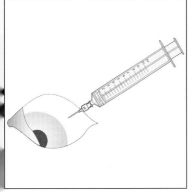

Fig 14.48 Injection into the vitreous body

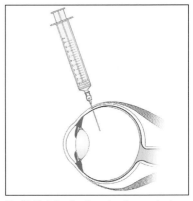

Fig 14.49 Injection into the vitreous body

Method

- **Preparation**
  - General anaesthesia

- **Technique**
  - Fixate the conjunctivae with a pair of atraumatic forceps
  - Puncture the anterior chamber from lateral and parallel to the iris
  - Aspirate chamber fluid
  - Exchange the syringe
  - Inject
  - Remove the needle and syringe

Complications

- Injury to the iris
- Infection
- Corneal oedema

15 Venous Access

Peripheral Venous Catheter

Indication

- Infusion/transfusion therapy
- Intravenous administration of medications

Peripheral Venous Catheter

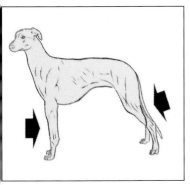

Fig 15.1 Venous access areas in the dog

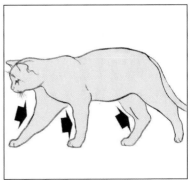

Fig 15.2 Venous access areas in the cat

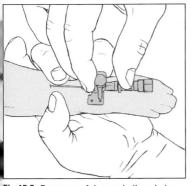

Fig 15.3 Puncture of the cephalic vein in the forelimb

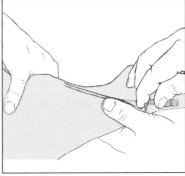

Fig 15.4 Puncture of the lateral saphenous vein in the dog

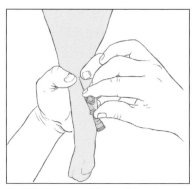

Fig 15.5 Puncture of the medial saphenous vein in the cat

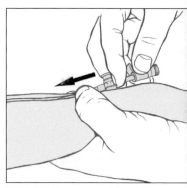

Fig 15.6 Advancement of the plastic catheter (method 1)

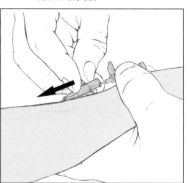

Fig 15.7 Advancement of the plastic catheter (method 2)

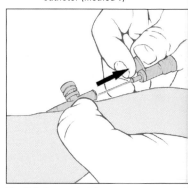

Fig 15.8 Removal of the steel stylet

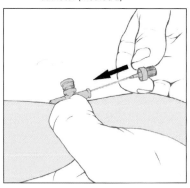

Fig 15.9 Attachment of a bung

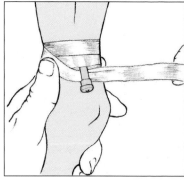

Fig 15.10 Dressing

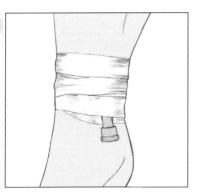

Fig 15.11 Dressing

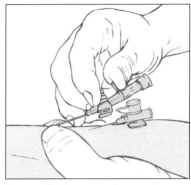

Fig 15.12 Further attempt in case of a malpuncture

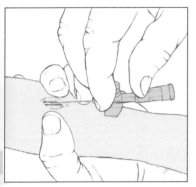

Fig 15.13 Venotomy

Method

- **Preparation**
  - Clip the fur and disinfect the skin
  - Sternal/prone position (cephalic vein), lateral recumbency (medial saphenous vein), standing (lateral saphenous vein)
  - Venous catheter in the dog (20 G pink or 18 G green)
  - Venous catheter in the cat (22 G blue or 24 G yellow)

  Venous puncture sites in the dog
  - Cephalic vein of the forelimb, lateral saphenous vein

  Venous puncture sites in the cat
  - Cephalic vein of the forelimb, medial saphenous vein

- **Technique**
  - Raise the vein (manually/tourniquet)
  - Puncture the skin and vein at about a 10° angle, until the incoming blood becomes visible in the base of the cannula
  - Withdraw the steel stylet

  One-hand-method (method 1)
  - Fixate the stylet with the thumb and fourth finger
  - Advance the plastic catheter with the fore and middle finger of the same hand

  Two-hand-method (method 2)
  - Fixate the stylet with the thumb and forefinger
  - Advance the plastic catheter with the thumb and forefinger of the other hand
  - Release the raised vein
  - Withdraw and remove the steel stylet
  - Attach a bung ± mandrel
  - Apply a dressing

Complications

- Paravasal malpuncture
- Collapse of the vein
- Thrombophlebitis
- Haematoma
- Abscess

Central Venous Catheter (CVC)

Indication

- Long term infusion therapy, chemotherapy, administration of hyperosmolar solutions
- Haemodynamic monitoring (measuring the central venous pressure)

Through-the-needle catheter

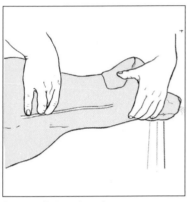

Fig 15.14 Raising the vein

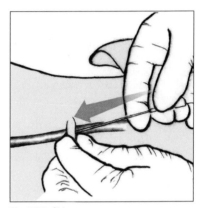

Fig 15.15 Skin puncture

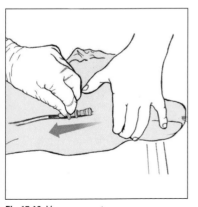

Fig 15.16 Venous puncture

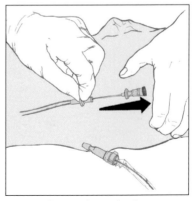

Fig 15.17 Remove the steel stylet

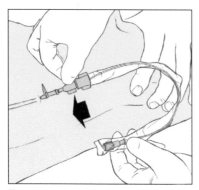

Fig 15.18 Attach the guidance sleeve onto the catheter

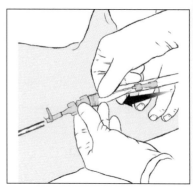

Fig 15.19 Insert the central venous catheter 'through the needle'

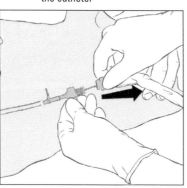

Fig 15.20 Release the guidance sleeve

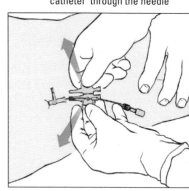

Fig 15.21 Divide and remove the guidance sleeve

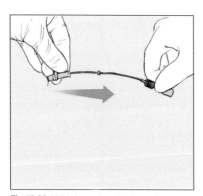

Fig 15.22 Withdraw the plastic catheter

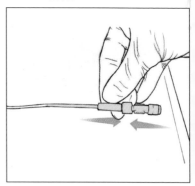

Fig 15.23 Screw the plastic catheter into the catheter base

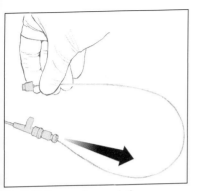

Fig 15.24 Remove the mandrel

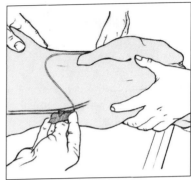

Fig 15.25 Apply a gauze swab with antibiotic cream

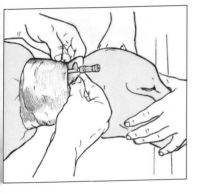

Fig 15.26 Dressing

Method

- **Preparation**
  - Clip the fur/disinfect the skin
  - Lateral recumbency
  - Venous catheter in the dog (Vygoflex Pur® 1.2 × 1.7mm, length 35mm [small dogs], 50mm [large dogs])
  - Venous catheter in the cat (Vygoflex Pur® 0.6 × 1.1mm, length 35mm)
  - Measure the length of the central venous catheter on the patient or an X-ray (puncture site to third intercostal space)

Venous puncture site
  - External jugular vein

- **Technique**
  - Manually raise the vein
  - Puncture the skin by lifting a skin fold and puncture the vein
  - Withdraw the steel stylet
  - Push the plastic catheter forwards
  - Release the raised vein
  - Remove the steel stylet
  - Attach the guidance sleeve to the end of the catheter
  - Insert the central venous catheter while in its protective sleeve up to the previously marked position
  - Release, divide and remove the guidance sleeve
  - Withdraw the plastic catheter and protective sleeve *very* carefully
  - Connect and screw the catheter into the catheter base
  - Take an X-ray to check the catheter is in the correct position (cranial vena cava, third intercostal space in front of the right atrium)
  - Perform an ECG
  - Remove the mandrel
  - Flush the central venous catheter (1,000 IE Heparin/500ml saline 0.9 per cent)
  - Attach injection caps
  - Apply a gauze swab with antibiotic cream (over puncture site)
  - Apply an adhesive dressing, with the catheter bandaged and fixated inside

Complications

- Atrial fibrillation
- Thrombophlebitis
- Air embolism
- Accidental removal/bending of the central venous catheter

Over-the-Wire Catheter (Seldinger technique)

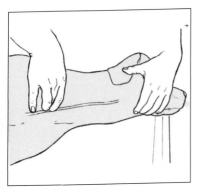

Fig 15.27 Raising of the vein

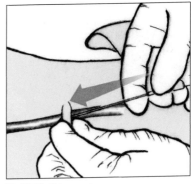

Fig 15.28 Skin puncture

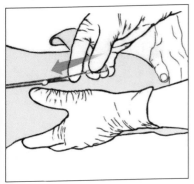

Fig 15.29 Venous puncture with an introducer needle

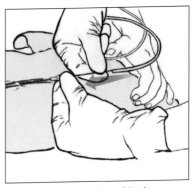

Fig 15.30 Insertion of the guidewire

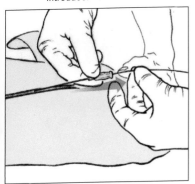

Fig 15.31 Removal of the steel stylet/ introducer needle

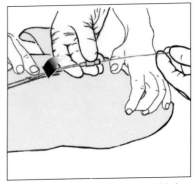

Fig 15.32 Widen the puncture site with the dilator

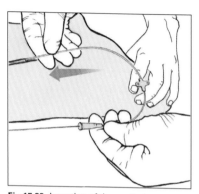

Fig 15.33 Insertion of the central venous catheter 'over-the-wire'

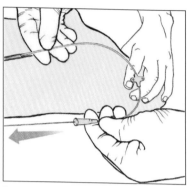

Fig 15.34 Removal of the guidewire

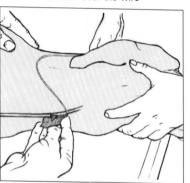

Fig 15.35 Gauze swab with antibiotic cream

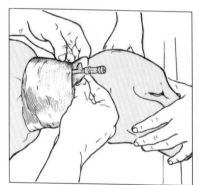

Fig 15.36 Dressing

Method

- **Preparation**
  - Clip the fur/disinfect the skin
  - Lateral recumbency
  - Venous catheter in the dog (Seldipur® 16 G, 30cm)
  - Measure the length of the central venous catheter on the patient or an X-ray (puncture site to third intercostal space)

Venous puncture site
  - External jugular vein

- **Technique**
  - Manually raise the vein
  - Puncture the skin by lifting a skin fold and puncture the vein
  - Withdraw the steel stylet
  - Advance a plastic catheter
  - Release the raised vein
  - Remove the steel stylet
  - Withdraw the wire inside the guidewire
  - Insert the wire and guidewire through the introducer needle into the vein
  - Remove the guidewire (while fixating the wire inside the venous lumen)
  - It may be necessary to widen the skin puncture site with a scalpel blade
  - Insert and remove the vessel dilator over the wire
  - Insert the central venous catheter over the wire up to the previously marked position
  - Remove the wire
  - Take an X-ray to check the catheter is in the correct position (cranial vena cava, third intercostal space in front of the right atrium)
  - Perform an ECG
  - Flush the central venous catheter (1,000 IE Heparin/500ml saline 0.9 per cent)
  - Attach injection caps
  - Apply gauze swab dressing with antibiotic cream over the puncture site
  - Apply an adhesive dressing, with the catheter bandaged and fixated inside

Complications

- Atrial fibrillation
- Thrombophlebitis
- Air embolism
- Accidental removal/bending of the central venous catheter

Venous catheter with a splittable cannula

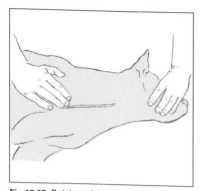

Fig 15.37 Raising of the vein

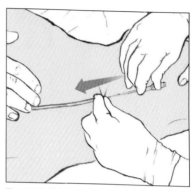

Fig 15.38 Skin puncture

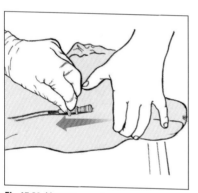

Fig 15.39 Venous puncture

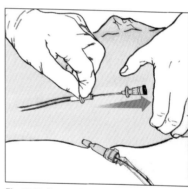

Fig 15.40 Removal of the steel stylet

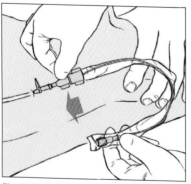

Fig 15.41 Attachment of the guidance sleeve

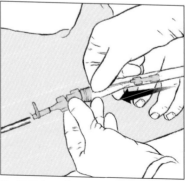

Fig 15.42 Insertion of the central venous catheter

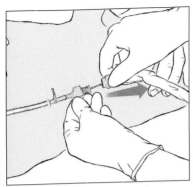

Fig 15.43 Release the guidance sleeve

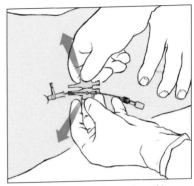

Fig 15.44 Divide and remove the guidance sleeve

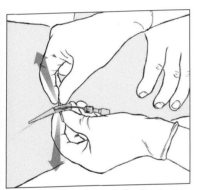

Fig 15.45 Withdraw and divide the plastic cannula

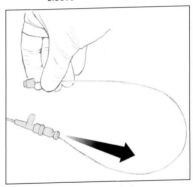

Fig 15.46 Remove the mandrel

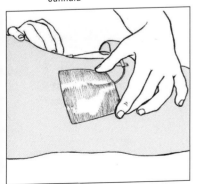

Fig 15.47 Apply a gauze swab with antibiotic cream

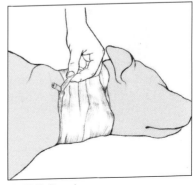

Fig 15.48 Dressing

Method

- **Preparation**
  - Clip the fur/disinfect the skin
  - Lateral recumbency
  - Venous catheter for the dog (Cavafix® Certo® with Splittocan® length 32 mm [small dogs], 45 mm [large dogs])
  - Measure the length of the central venous catheter on the patient or an X-ray (puncture site to third intercostal space)

  Venous puncture site
  - External jugular vein

- **Technique**
  - Manually raise the vein
  - Puncture the skin by lifting a skin fold and puncture the vein
  - Withdraw the stylet
  - Advance the plastic catheter
  - Release the raised vein
  - Remove the stylet
  - Attach the guidance sleeve onto the end of the plastic catheter
  - Insert the central venous catheter while in its protective sleeve up to the marked position
  - Remove the push-on contact (red) and protective sleeve
  - Release, divide and remove the guidance sleeve
  - Withdraw, divide and remove the plastic catheter from inside the vein
  - Take an X-ray to check the catheter is in the correct position (cranial vena cava, third intercostal space in front of the right atrium)
  - Perform an ECG
  - Remove the mandrel
  - Flush the central venous catheter (1,000 IE Heparin/500ml saline 0.9 per cent)
  - Attach an injection cap
  - Apply a gauze swab with antibiotic cream to the puncture site
  - Apply an adhesive dressing adhesive, with the catheter bandaged and fixated inside

Complications

- Atrial fibrillation
- Thrombophlebitis
- Air embolism
- Accidental removal/bending of the central venous catheter

Venotomy

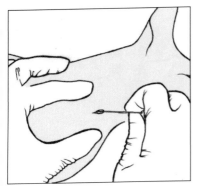

Fig 15.49 Skin incision

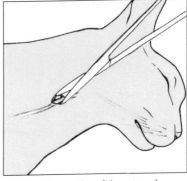

Fig 15.50 Preparation of the external jugular vein

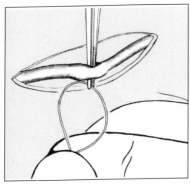

Fig 15.51 Placement of stay sutures

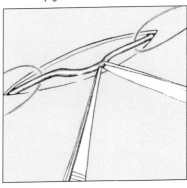

Fig 15.52 Venotomy

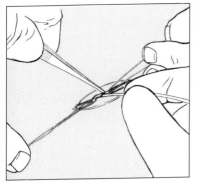

Fig 15.53 Insertion of the central venous catheter

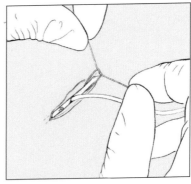

Fig 15.54 Vessel ligatures

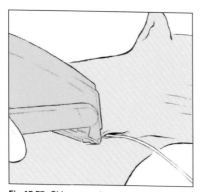

Fig 15.55 Skin suture/staples

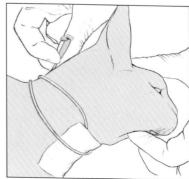

Fig 15.56 Apply a gauze swab with antibiotic cream

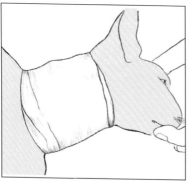

Fig 15.57 Dressing

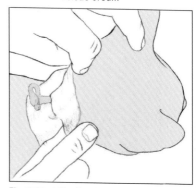

Fig 15.58 Adhesive dressing (inside) for the fixation of the catheter

Method

- **Preparation**
  - Clip the fur/disinfect the skin
  - Lateral recumbency
  - Venous catheter in the cat
  - Measure the length of the central venous catheter on the patient or an X-ray (puncture site to third intercostal space)

Venotomy Site: External Jugular Vein

- **Technique**
  - Manually raise the vein
  - Make a paravascular skin incision with a scalpel blade
  - Prepare the external jugular vein
  - Place two stay sutures (absorbable sutures [2–0])
  - Perform a venotomy with a pair of forceps and Metzenbaum scissors
  - Release the raised vein
  - Insert the central venous catheter up to the marked position
  - Tighten the vessel ligatures (first distal, then proximal over the catheter)
  - Take an X-ray to check the catheter is in the correct position (cranial vena cava, third intercostal space in front of the right atrium)
  - Perform an ECG
  - Flush the central venous catheter (1,000 IE Heparin/500ml saline 0.9 per cent)
  - Attach an injection cap
  - Suture or staple the skin
  - Apply a gauze swab with antibiotic cream over the puncture site
  - Adhesive dressing with the catheter carefully bandaged and fixated inside

Complications

- Atrial fibrillation
- Thrombophlebitis
- Air embolism
- Accidental removal/bending of the central venous catheter
- Strangulation by the venous catheter, which is wrapped around the neck

Intraosseal Access

Indication

- Emergency infusion therapy/transfusion therapy when no venous access is available (especially in neonatal intensive care medicine)

Intraosseal Access

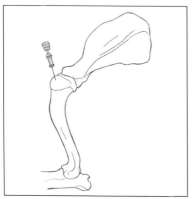

Fig 15.59 Puncture site of the humerus

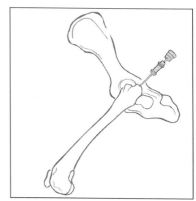

Fig 15.60 Puncture site of the femur

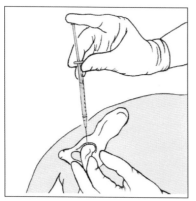

Fig 15.61 Topical anaesthesia

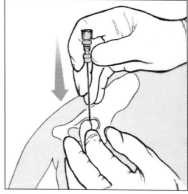

Fig 15.62 Soft tissue puncture/localisation of the trochanteric fossa

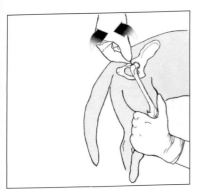

Fig 15.63 Screwing the puncture needle into the bone

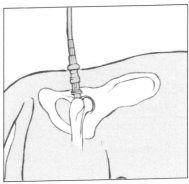

Fig 15.64 Attachment of the infusion line

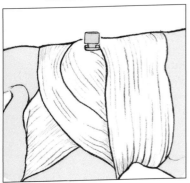

Fig 15.65 Dressing

Method

- **Preparation**
  - Clip the fur/disinfect the skin
  - Lateral recumbency
  - Topical anaesthesia (lidocaine 1 per cent): periosteal infiltration
  - Puncture needle (Spinal needle, 1.3 × 75mm bone marrow needle (Rosenthal needle)

Access sites
  - Trochanteric fossa of the femur

- **Technique**
  - Fixate the hind limb
  - Puncture the skin with the puncture needle placed in the trochanteric fossa of the femur
  - Screw the puncture needle/bone marrow needle into the femur along its vertical axis
  - Remove the mandrel
  - Flush the catheter with saline
  - Attach an injection cap or the infusion line
  - Apply a swab gauze with antibiotic cream to the puncture site
  - Apply a cotton and elastic gauze dressing

Complications

- Osteomyelitis
- Septicaemia
- Air embolism

16 Infusion

Intravenous Infusion (gravity assisted)

Indication

- Fluid therapy

Intravenous Infusion (gravity assisted)

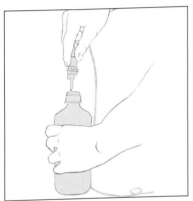

Fig 16.1 Pierce the rubber membrane

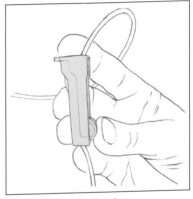

Fig 16.2 Close the roller clamp

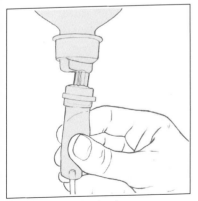

Fig 16.3 Fill the drip chamber

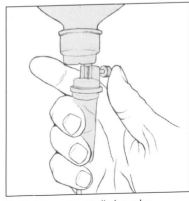

Fig 16.4 Open the ventilation valve

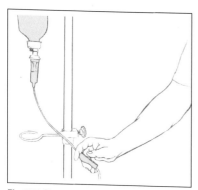

Fig 16.5 Remove all air from the infusion line

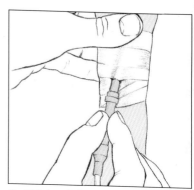

Fig 16.6 Attach the infusion line

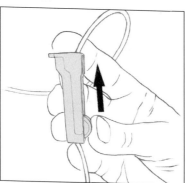

Fig 16.7 Open the roller clamp

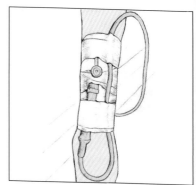

Fig 16.8 Fixation of the infusion line

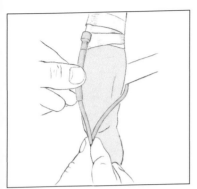

Fig 16.9 Flushing of the venous catheter
(infusion line)

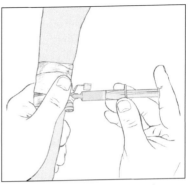

Fig 16.10 Flushing of the venous catheter
(injection port)

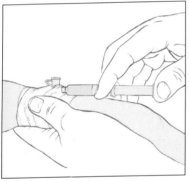

Fig 16.11 Flushing of the venous catheter
(infusion port)

Method

- **Preparation**
    - Calculate the infusion volume and rate
    - Maximum infusion rate (peripheral venous catheter)
    - 22 G (blue)   25ml/min
    - 20 G (rose)   55ml/min
    - 18 G (green)   90ml/min
    - Infuse bodywarm infusion solution

- **Technique**
    - Pierce the rubber membrane on the bottle with the spike on the infusion line
    - Close the roller clamp
    - Attach the infusion bottle to the infusion stand (height regulation about 30cm)
    - Fill the drip chamber (c. 1/3)
    - Open the ventilation valve
    - Remove all air in the infusion line over a sink by opening the roller clamp and closing it again once no air bubbles are left
    - Attach infusion line to venous catheter
    - Open the roller clamp and set the infusion rate
    - Fixate the infusion line

Flushing a blocked infusion line

1. Bend the infusion line and press the rubber cuff several times
2. Inject 5ml of the infusion solution into the injection or infusion port of the venous catheter

Complications

- Thrombophlebitis

Subcutaneous Infusion Therapy

Indication

- Subcutaneous depot infusion

Subcutaneous infusion (gravity assisted)

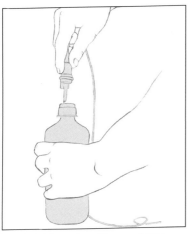

Fig 16.12 Pierce the rubber membrane

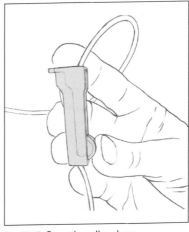

Fig 16.13 Open the roller clamp

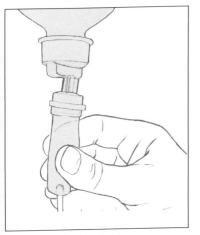

Fig 16.14 Fill the drip chamber

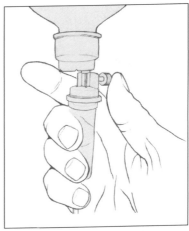

Fig 16.15 Open the ventilation valve

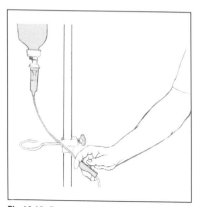

Fig 16.16 Remove all air from the infusion line

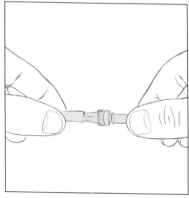

Fig 16.17 Attach a hypodermic needle to the infusion line

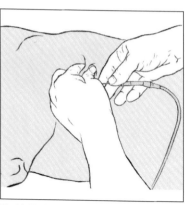

Fig 16.18 Skin puncture

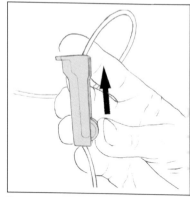

Fig 16.19 Open the roller clamp

Method

- **Preparation**
  - Calculate the infusion volume (about 100ml)
  - Depot infusion of bodywarm infusion solutions
  - No hyperosmolar solutions (glucose solutions)

- **Technique**
  - Pierce the rubber membrane of the bottle with the spike of the infusion line
  - Close the roller clamp
  - Attach the infusion bottle to an infusion stand (height regulation c. 30cm)
  - Fill the drip chamber (c. 1/3)
  - Open the ventilation valve
  - Remove all air from the infusion line over a sink by opening the roller clamp and closing it again once all air has been removed
  - Attach a hypodermic needle (20G yellow)
  - Skin puncture (see subcutaneous injection)
  - Open the roller clamp
  - Infusion
  - Close the roller clamp
  - Remove the hypodermic needle
  - Compress the puncture site

Complications

- Painfulness
- Necrosis
- Slow absorption

Infusion Pump

Indication

- Regulation of the infusion rate during intravenous, gravity assisted infusion

Infusion Pump

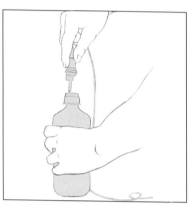

Fig 16.20 Pierce the rubber membrane

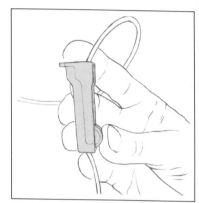

Fig 16.21 Close the roller clamp

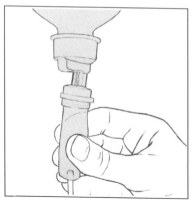

Fig 16.22 Fill the drip chamber

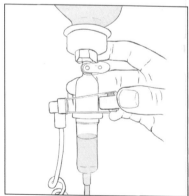

Fig 16.23 Attach the droplet sensor

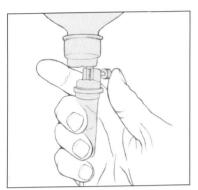

Fig 16.24 Open the ventilation valve

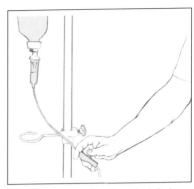

Fig 16.25 Remove all air from the infusion line

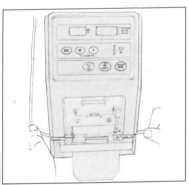

Fig 16.26 Place the infusion line into the pump

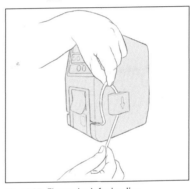

Fig 16.27 Fixate the infusion line

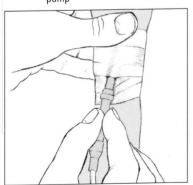

Fig 16.28 Attach the infusion line

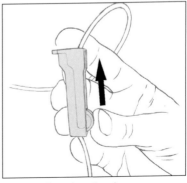

Fig 16.29 Open the roller clamp

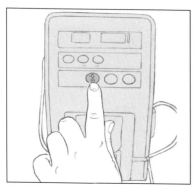

Fig 16.30 Switch the pump on

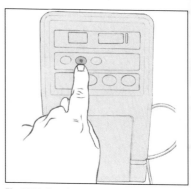

Fig 16.31 Set the infusion rate

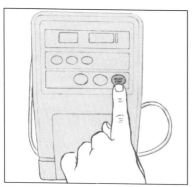

Fig 16.32 Press 'start' button

Method

- **Preparation**
    - Calculate the infusion volume and rate
    - Maximum infusion rate (peripheral venous catheter)
    - 22 G (blue)   25ml/min
    - 20 G (pink)   55ml/min
    - 18 G (green) 90ml/min
    - Infuse body warm infusion solutions
    - System: MCM 404®, Fresenius Vial

- **Technique**
    - Pierce the rubber membrane of the infusion bottle with the spike of the infusion line
    - Close the roller clamp
    - Attach the infusion bottle onto the infusion stand (height regulation about 30cm)
    - Fill the drip chamber (c. 1/3)
    - Open the ventilation valve
    - Remove all air from the infusion line over a sink by opening the roller clamp and closing it again once all air bubbles have been removed
    - Open the lid on the infusion pump, put the infusion line inside and fixate it at the side of the pump
    - Attach the infusion line to the venous catheter
    - Open the rolling clamp
    - Switch the pump on
    - Set the infusion rate
    - Press 'start'
    - Fixate the infusion line

Complications

- Bending of the infusion line

Syringe Driver

Indication

- Intravenous pressure infusion of medications (mannitol, dopamine, dobutamine, lidocaine, propofol, diazepam, diltiazem, fentanyl, insulin, isoproterenol)

Syringe Driver

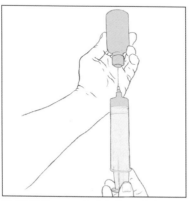

Fig 16.33 Draw up the infusion solution

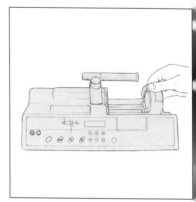

Fig 16.34 Pull the actuator out

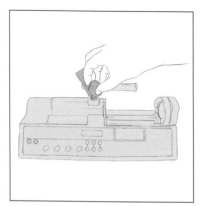

Fig 16.35 Open the barrel clamp arm

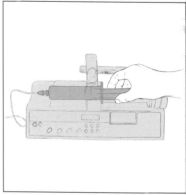

Fig 16.36 Insert the infusion syringe

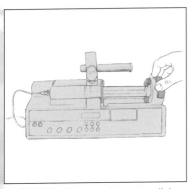

Fig 16.37 The plunger and actuator click into place

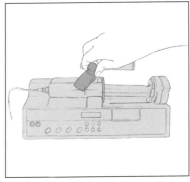

Fig 16.38 Close the barrel clamp arm

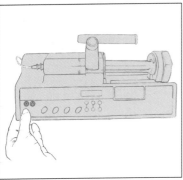

Fig 16.39 Switch the syringe driver on

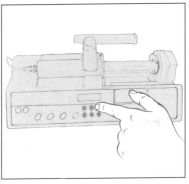

Fig 16.40 Set the infusion rate

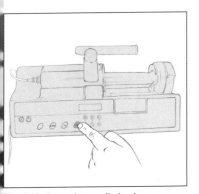

Fig 16.41 Press the ventilation button

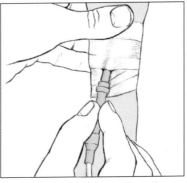

Fig 16.42 Attach the infusion line to the patient

Method

- **Preparation**
    - Calculate the drug's dilution factor, infusion rate and volume
    - Possibly dilute the infusion solution
    - Infuse body warm infusion solutions
    - System: Pilot A2®, Fresenius Vial, infusion syringe 50ml

- **Technique**
    - Draw up the infusion solution into the infusion syringe
    - Attach the infusion line to the syringe
    - Unlock and pull out the actuator
    - Open the barrel clamp arm on the syringe driver
    - Insert the infusion syringe
    - The actuator clicks into place
    - Close the barrel clamp arm
    - Switch the syringe driver on
    - Set the infusion rate and volume
    - Press the bolus button (it automatically removes the air from the infusion line)
    - Attach the infusion line to the venous catheter
    - Press the 'start' button

Complications

- Overinfusion

17 Transfusion

Full Blood Transfusion

Indication

- Anaemia, thrombocytopenia, plasmatic coagulopathy

Full Blood Transfusion in the dog

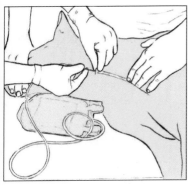

Fig 17.1 Skin puncture

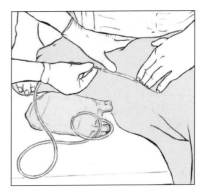

Fig 17.2 Puncture of the external jugular vein

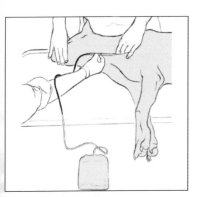

Fig 17.3 Blood collection

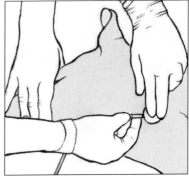

Fig 17.4 Removal of the puncture needle

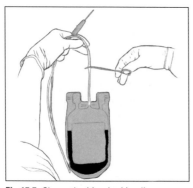

Fig 17.5 Clamp the blood taking line

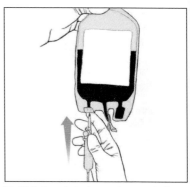

Fig 17.6 Attach the bag to the transfusion line

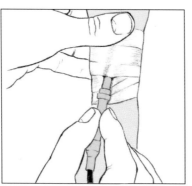

Fig 17.7 Connect the transfusion line

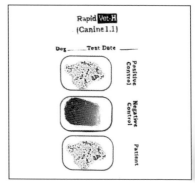

Fig 17.8 Blood typing (DEA-1.1) (Rapid Vet-H® canine test cards)

Method

- **System**
  - Standard closed blood collection systems, multibag systems

- **Donor suitability**
  - > 30kg
  - Young
  - Healthy
  - Good tempered
  - DEA-1.1/1.2/7 neg
  - Brucella–, ehrlichia–, leishmania–, babesia–, dirofilaria– neg.
  - No self-transfusion (as recipient)

- **Transfusion volume**
  - Volume (ml) = 85 (dog) or 60 (cat) × BW (kg) × [(Desired PCV – Actual PCV)/Donor PCV]
  - dog = 10–20ml/kg BW (donor) (usually 450–500ml/dog > 25kg broadly correct (BW)

- **Anticoagulant**
  - If full blood collection < 450ml remove a proportional and sterile amount of CPDA-1 (anticoagulant solution) out of the transfusion bag
  - 70ml CPDA-1/500ml full blood

- **Blood collection**
  - Intravenous infusion access (peripheral venous catheter) (donor)
  - Hold the donor in lateral recumbency with an extended neck (possibly slight sedation)
  - Clip the fur
  - Disinfect the skin
  - Raise the vein
  - Indirect puncture of the external jugular vein
    1. Elevate a skin fold
    2. Puncture the skin
    3. Puncture the vein
  - Fixate the puncture needle during the blood collection
  - At the end of the collection remove the puncture needle and apply pressure over the puncture site with a gauze swab (compression time about 2–3 min)
  - Clamp, knot and cut the collection line tubing

- **Infusion**
  - Full electrolyte solution (twice the amount of blood lost) (donor)

- **Cross matching**
  - No adverse reactions to be expected in first time recipients of unrelated donors

Blood typing (DEA-1.1) (Rapid Vet-H® canine test cards)
  - Collect at least 0.5ml EDTA blood
  - Label the test card
  - Apply one drop of diluent solution into each test well
  - Add one drop of positive control solution into the DEA-1.1 positive control well
  - Mix the solution with the spatula contained in test kit

- Add 1 drop of negative control solution into DEA-1.1 negative control well
- Mix the solution with the spatula contained in test kit
- Swill the EDTA blood sample
- Pipette and add one drop of the blood sample into the patient test well
- Mix the blood sample with a new spatula included in the test kit
- Swill the test card horizontally (about 2 min)
- Position the test card in an angle of 30–45°
- Read the test results, example:
  - 1. Positive control (agglutination)
  - 2. Negative control (no agglutination)
  - 3. Patient (agglutination = DEA 1.1 positive): i.e. suitable as recipient of DEA-1.1-positive and DEA-1.1-negative blood *and* no suitability as blood donor for DEA-1.1-negative recipients

Cross matching test (major test/minor test)
- Take a blood sample and fill an EDTA and serum tube each from both the recipient and donor
- Centrifuge the serum tubes (donor and recipient serum)
- Wash the erythrocytes of the EDTA tubes (donor and recipient erythrocytes) (centrifuge, decant the plasma, fill the tubes with saline, centrifuge, decant the plasma)
- Make a 4 per cent cell suspension (donor and recipient tube) (0.2ml washed erythrocytes + 4.8ml saline)
- Label the test tubes

Major test
- Two drops (0.1ml) donor cell suspension + 2 drops (0.1ml) recipient serum

Minor Test
- Two drops (0.1ml) donor serum + two drops (0.1ml) recipient cell suspension

Donor control test
- 2 drops (0.1ml) donor cell suspension + two drops (0.1ml) donor serum

Recipient control test
- Two drops (0.1ml) recipient cell suspension + two drops (0.1ml) recipient serum

- Incubate the test tubes for 15 min at room temperature (ideally 37°C, 25°C and 4°C)
- Centrifuge the test tubes at 1000 RPM for about 1 min
- Read the test results
  1. Donor control (no agglutination)
  2. Recipient control (no agglutination)
  3. Major test (agglutination = incompatible)
  4. Minor test (agglutination = partially incompatible) (transfusion possibly based on clinical judgement in the absence of an alternative donor)

- **Transfusion**
  - Attach the transfusion line including a micropore filter (recipient) to the transfusion bag and intravenous catheter
  - Initial transfusion rate 0.25ml/kg/h for about 15 min, then 10ml/kg/h (max. 4ml/kg/h in patients with cardiac insufficiency)

Complications

- **Acute haemolysis**
  - With DEA-1.1/1.2 positive donor and DEA-1.1/1.2 (transfusion)
  - Negative recipient with previous sensitisation
  - Principal symptoms: haemoglobinaemia/-uria, excitation, tachycardia, renal failure, anaphylaxis, urticaria
  - Therapy: stop the transfusion, give glucocorticoid, infusion of a full electrolyte solution
  - Delayed haemolysis with DEA 3,5,7 incompatibility

- **Anaphylaxis**
  - Membrane bound antigen incompatibilities, anticoagulant incompatibilities
  - Principal symptoms: urticaria, fever, shock
  - Therapy: stop the transfusion, give adrenaline, glucocorticoids, infusion of a full electrolyte solution

- **Volume overload**
  - Principal symptoms: cough, tachypnoea, vomitus, pulmonary oedema
  - Therapy: stop the transfusion, commence diuresis

Full Blood Transfusion in the cat

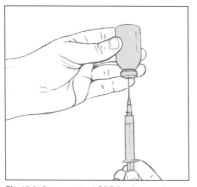

Fig 17.9 Draw up 7ml CPDA-1 in a syringe

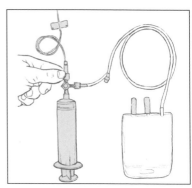

Fig 17.10 Attach a butterfly catheter

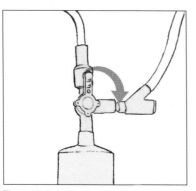

Fig 17.11 Open the three-way tap

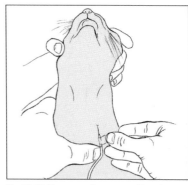

Fig 17.12 Puncture the external jugular vein

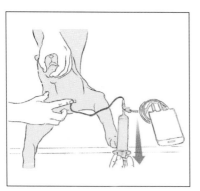

Fig 17.13 Blood collections (50ml) while slightly aspirating

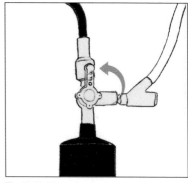

Fig 17.14 Close the three-way tap

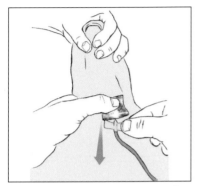

Fig 17.15 Removal of the puncture needle

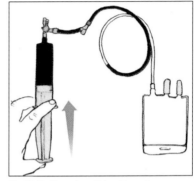

Fig 17.16 Transfer of blood into the transfusion bag

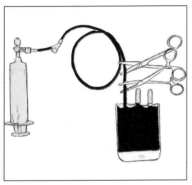

Fig 17.17 Clamp/cut off the collection line

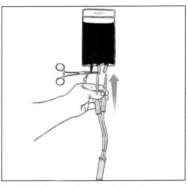

Fig 17.18 Attach the transfusion line (including filter)

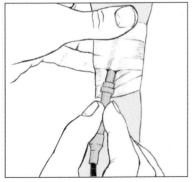

Fig 17.19 Attach transfusion line to intravenous catheter

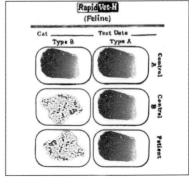

Fig 17.20 Blood typing (A, B, AB)

- **System**
  - Transfusion Set

- **Suitability as donor**
  - > 4.5kg
  - Young
  - Healthy
  - Good tempered
  - Compatible blood type: blood type A to blood type A and blood type AB, blood type B to blood type B
  - FeLV-, FIV-, FIP- and hemobartonella-neg
  - No previous transfusion (as recipient)

- **Transfusion volume**
  - ml required to raise haematocrit by 1 per cent (recipient) = 2.2ml full blood × kg BW
  - Desired haematocrit change (recipient)
  - Haematocrit (donor)

- **Transfusion volume**
  - Cat = 10ml/kg BW (usually 50ml/cat > 5 kg BW) (donor)

- **Anticoagulant**
  - 7ml CPDA-1/50ml full blood
  - Remove the three-way tap from the syringe
  - Attach the needle to the syringe
  - Draw up 7ml CPDA-1 into the syringe
  - Remove the needle and attach the three-way tap

- **Blood collection**
  - Hold the donor in sternal/prone position with an extended neck (donor) (possibly slight sedation)
  - Clip the fur
  - Disinfect the skin
  - Raise the vein
  - Direct puncture of the external jugular vein with a butterfly catheter
  - Manually fixate the butterfly during the blood collection
  - Collect 50ml of blood while slightly aspirating with a syringe
  - Close the three-way tap at the end of the blood collection
  - Remove the puncture needle while compressing the puncture site with a gauze swab (compression time about 2–3 min)
  - Remove the collection line from the three-way tap
  - Swill the syringe (mix the blood/anticoagulant)

- Transfer the blood from the syringe into the transfusion bag (by injection)
- Clamp (mosquito forceps) and cut off the transfusion line (from the syringe to transfusion bag)

- **Infusion (donor)**
  - Subcutaneous depot infusion (twice the amount of blood lost)

- **Cross matching**
  - Blood Typing (A, B, AB) (Rapid Vet-H® feline test cards)
  - Collect at least 0.5ml EDTA blood
  - Label the test card
  - Apply one drop of the diluent solution into each test well
  - Add one drop each of the control-A solution into the control-A/type-A well and control-A/type-B well
  - Mix the solution with the spatula included in the test kit
  - Add one drop each of the control-B solution into the control-B/type-A well and control-B/type-B well
  - Mix the solution with a new spatula included in the test kit
  - Swill the EDTA blood sample, pipette one drop of blood each into the patient/type-A well and patient/type-B well
  - Mix the solution with a new spatula included in the test kit
  - Swill the test card horizontally for about 2 min
  - Position the test card in a 30–45° angle
  - Read the test results
    1. Agglutination in patient/type-A well (patient blood group A), i.e., suitability as donor for blood group A and possibly blood group AB
    2. Agglutination in patient/type-B well (patient blood group B), i.e., suitability as donor for blood group B and possibly blood group AB
    3. Agglutination in patient/type-A well and patient/type-B well (patient blood group AB), i.e., suitability as donor for blood group AB

Cross matching (major test / minor test)
- Take a blood sample and fill an EDTA and serum tube each from both the recipient and donor
- Centrifuge the serum tubes (donor and recipient serum)
- Wash the erythrocytes of the EDTA tubes three times (donor and recipient erythrocytes) (centrifuge, decant the plasma, fill the tubes with saline, centrifuge, decant the plasma)

- Make a 4 per cent cell suspension (donor and recipient tube) (0.2ml washed erythrocytes + 4.8ml saline)
- Label the test tubes

Major test
- Two drops (0.1ml) donor cell suspension + two drops (0.1ml) recipient serum

Minor test
- Two drops (0.1ml) donor serum + two drops (0.1ml) recipient cell suspension

Donor control test
- Two drops (0.1ml) donor cell suspension + two drops (0.1ml) donor serum

Recipient control test
- Two drops (0.1ml) recipient cell suspension + two drops (0.1ml) recipient serum
- Incubate the test tubes for 15 mins at room temperature (ideally 37°C, 25°C and 4°C)
- Centrifuge the test tubes at 1,000 RPM for about 1 min
- Read the test results
    1. Donor control (no agglutination)
    2. Recipient control (no agglutination)
    3. Major test (agglutination = incompatible)
    4. Minor test (agglutination = partially incompatible) (transfusion possibly based on clinical judgement in the absence of an alternative donor)

- **Transfusion**
    - Attach the transfusion line including a micropore filter (recipient) to the transfusion bag and intravenous catheter
    - Initial transfusion rate 0.25ml/kg/h for about 15 min, then 10ml/kg/h (max. 4ml/kg/h in patients with cardiac insufficiency)

Complications

- **Acute haemolysis**
    - With blood group A donor and blood group B donor
    - Principal symptoms: haemoglobinaemia/-uria, excitation, tachycardia, renal failure, anaphylaxis, urticaria
    - Therapy: stop the transfusion, give glucocorticoids, commence infusion of a full electrolyte solution

- **Anaphylaxis**
  - Membrane bound antigen incompatibilities, anticoagulant incompatibilities
  - Principal symptoms: urticaria, fever, shock
  - Therapy: stop the transfusion, give adrenaline, glucocorticoids, infusion (full electrolyte solution)

- **Volume overload**
  - Principal symptoms: cough, tachypnoea, vomitus, pulmonary oedema
  - Therapy: stop the transfusion, commence diuresis

Preparation of Preserved Blood Units

Indication

- Erythrocyte concentrate (anaemia)
  - Plasma (plasmatic coagulopathies, acute pancreatitis)

Plasma Production

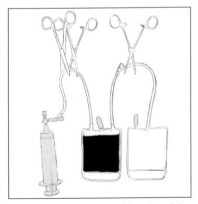

Fig 17.21 Multibag system (clamping of the lines)

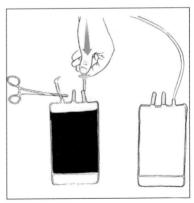

Fig 17.22 Transfusion bag (attach to transfer bag)

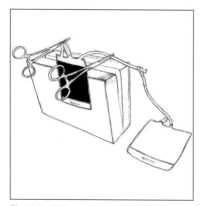

Fig 17.23 Fridge storage for 8–12 hours

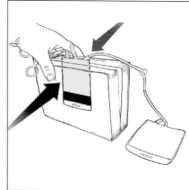

Fig 17.24 Plasma transfer

- **System**
  - Multibag system
  - Transfer bag

- **Preparation**

  Multibag system
  - Clamp (mosquito forceps), cut and remove the blood collection line (from the syringe or puncture needle to the transfusion bag)
  - Clamp (mosquito forceps) the transfer line (from the transfusion to the transfer bag)

  Transfusion bag system
  - Clamp (mosquito forceps), cut and remove the blood collection line (from the puncture needle to the transfusion bag)
  - Connect to the transfer bag
  - Clamp (mosquito forceps)

  the transfer line (from the transfusion bag to the transfer bag)

- **Technique**
  - Store in a fridge inside a large book to promote sedimentation (8–12 hours)
  - Open the mosquito forceps
  - Close the book under gentle pressure (transfer about 80 per cent of the plasma into the transfer bag)
  - Clamp and seal each side of the transfer line

- **Storage**
  - Plasma (freezer at –30°C keeps up to 12 months)
  - Erythrocyte concentrate (immediate transfusion or preparation with ADSOL preservative solution and storage up to one month at 4°C)

Autotransfusion

Indication

- Emergency measure in case of dicoumarol poisoning, haemothorax and anaemia

Autotransfusion

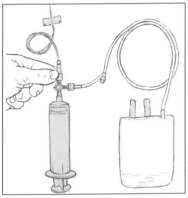

Fig 17.25 Transfusion set

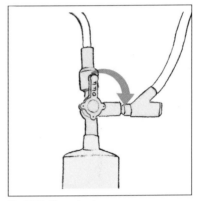

Fig 17.26 Open the three-way tap

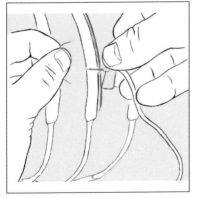

Fig 17.27 Thorax puncture (6–7 ICR)

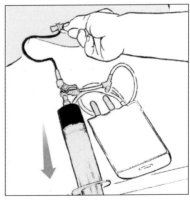

Fig 17.28 Thorax drainage

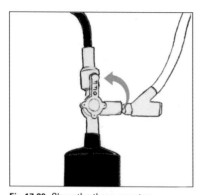

Fig 17.29 Close the three-way tap

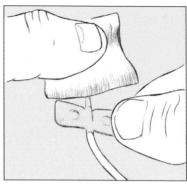

Fig 17.30 Remove the butterfly catheter and apply compression

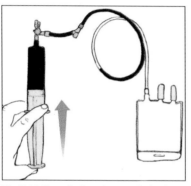

Fig 17.31 Transfer into the transfusion bag

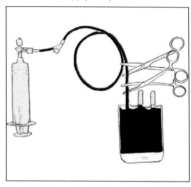

Fig 17.32 Clamping/cutting of the collection line

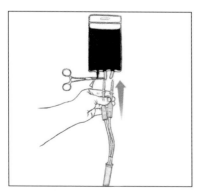

Fig 17.33 Attach the transfusion line (including filter)

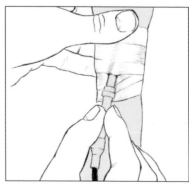

Fig 17.34 Connect the transfusion line to the patient

Method

- **Preparation**
  - System: standard transfusion set
  - Position of patient: lying (sternal/prone position)/standing
  - Clip the fur/disinfect the skin

- **Technique**

  ### Thorax puncture
  - Sixth–seventh intercostal space, lower third, cranial to the rib
  - Lift the skin towards rostral at the puncture site
  - Position the three-way tap (horizontal = open towards syringe)
  - Puncture the thorax with a butterfly catheter while slightly aspirating
  - Drain the thorax /aspirate into the syringe
  - Close the three-way tap = open towards the transfusion bag
  - Remove the butterfly catheter while compressing the puncture site with a gauze swab for about 5 min

  ### Blood transfer
  - Inject the blood into the transfer bag
  - Clamp, cut off and remove the collection line (from the syringe to the transfusion bag)

  ### Transfusion
  - Connect the transfusion line including a micropore filter to the transfusion bag and intravenous catheter
  - Autotransfusion rate: 10–20ml/kg/h

Complications

- Thromboembolism
- Perforation of the lung
- Damage to the rib vessels
- Pneumothorax
- Infection

18 Inhalation

Oxygen Supplementation

Indication

- Inhalation of oxygen and inhalation anaesthetics
- Inhalation of medicines (antibiotics, antimycotics, cortisone preparations et al)

Oxygen Supplementation

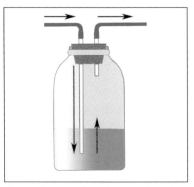

Fig 18.1 Pressure flow of oxygen through water

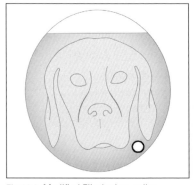

Fig 18.2 Modified Elizabethan collar

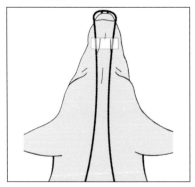

Fig 18.3 Nasal cannula

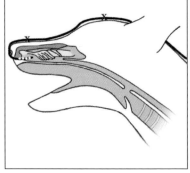

Fig 18.4 Nasal probe

Method

- **Technique**

    ### Oxygen cage/tent
    - Commercial systems, e.g., Shor-Line®, neonatal incubators (human medicine)
    - Requires oxygen humidification via pressure feeding through saline
    - Oxygen flow rate 2–4 l/min.

    ### Modified Elizabethan collar
    - Cover the cone to about 90 per cent with cling film and supply oxygen through the attachment at the collar
    - Oxygen flow rate 4–6–8 l/min.

    ### Nasal cannula
    - Commercial systems from humane medicine are suitable for large dogs
    - Fixation on the skin via skin sutures/superglue or over the bridge of the nose with adhesive tape
    - Requires oxygen humidification via pressure feeding through saline
    - Elizabethan collar essential
    - Oxygen flow rate 4–6 l/min.

    ### Nasal probe/tube
    - Human neonatal feeding tubes (4–8FR)
    - Intranasal application of lidocaine 2 per cent solution
    - Raise the head (1–2 min)
    - Moisturise the tube with lubricant and lidocaine
    - Insert the tube into the ventral nasal meatus (up to about fourth premolar)
    - Fixate the tube with skin sutures/superglue lateral to the nostril and forehead
    - Requires oxygen humidification via pressure feeding through saline
    - Elizabethan collar essential
    - Oxygen flow rate 4–8 l/min.

Complications

- Dehydration/irritation of the airways
- Epistaxis

Endotracheal Intubation

Indication

- Oxygen supplementation/inhalation anaesthesia
- Ventilation

Endotracheal Intubation

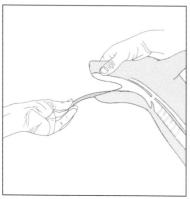

Fig 18.5 Pull out the tongue

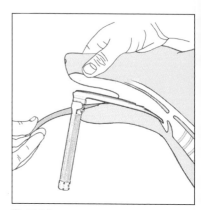

Fig 18.6 Laryngoscopy

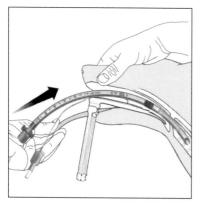

Fig 18.7 Endotracheal insertion of the endotracheal (ET) tube

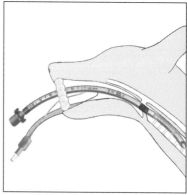

Fig 18.8 Insert a mouth wedge

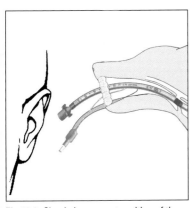

Fig 18.9 Check the correct position of the ET tube via auscultation

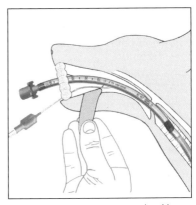

Fig 18.10 Pull the tongue out to the side

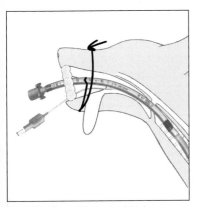

Fig 18.11 Tie and fixate the ET tube

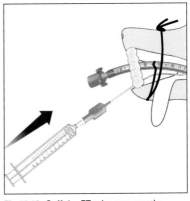

Fig 18.12 Cuff the ET tube very gently

Method

- **Preparation**
  - Sedation
  - Sternal position/lateral recumbency/dorsal position
  - Choice of ET tube: as big as possible, easy to insert, measure the ET tube length on the patient
  - ET tube preparation: fixate the ties, check the patency of the ET tube, check the cuff, moisten the ET tube with water
  - Topical anaesthesia of the larynx (Lidocaine 2 per cent spray) especially in cats

- **Technique**
  - Hold the patient with the neck extended, pull out the tongue with a gauze swab
  - Perform laryngoscopy and press down the tongue (without touching the glottis)
  - Gently insert the ET tube (possibly including a guidance rod) over the laryngoscope (during inspiration)
  - Place the mouth wedge and pull the tongue out to the side
  - Check the correct position of the ET tube (audible breathing sounds, palpable breath at the tube outlet)
  - Fixate the ET tube
  - Dog (mandibular, then maxillary loop tie)
  - Cat (mandibular loop tie, then loop tie behind the ears)
  - Slowly and gently cuff the ET tube

Complications

- Laryngospasm
- Tracheal rupture
- Unilateral lung ventilation

Emergency Intubation (Seldinger technique)

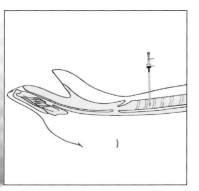

Fig 18.13 Tracheal puncture

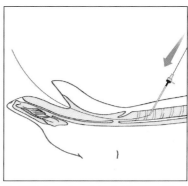

Fig 18.14 Insertion of the Seldinger guide wire

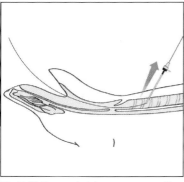

Fig 18.15 Removal of the puncture needle

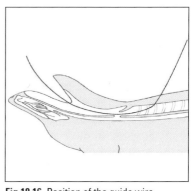

Fig 18.16 Position of the guide wire

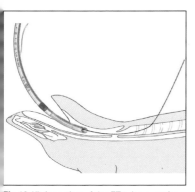

Fig 18.17 Insertion of the ET tube over the guide wire

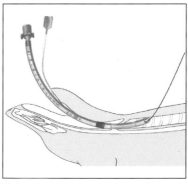

Fig 18.18 Removal of the guide wire

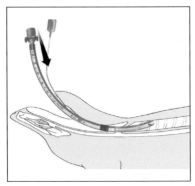

Fig 18.19 Continued insertion of the ET tube

Method

- **Preparation**
  - Sedation
  - Dorsal position/lateral recumbency
  - Clip the fur, disinfect the skin
  - Topical anaesthesia of the larynx (Lidocaine 2 per cent spray) especially in cats
  - System: central venous catheter set

- **Technique**
  - Transcutaneous tracheal puncture with a cannula (second–fourth tracheal ring) (Seldinger technique)
  - Insert the Seldinger guide wire (from the CVC set) through the cannula into the tracheal lumen
  - Advance the guide wire towards rostral/cranial, until it becomes visible in the oral cavity
  - Endotracheal insertion of the ET tube over the guide wire
  - Remove the guide wire
  - Advance the ET tube

Complications

- Glottal oedema
- Subcutaneous emphysema
- Infection

Tracheotomy

Indication

- Tracheal obstruction (foreign body, tumour, glottal oedema, laryngeal trauma)

Tracheotomy

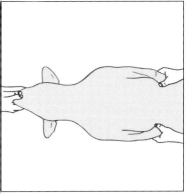

Fig 18.20 Position for tracheotomy

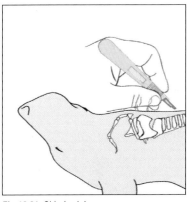

Fig 18.21 Skin incision

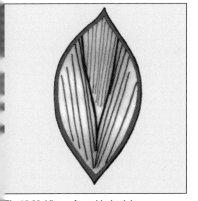

Fig 18.22 View after skin incision

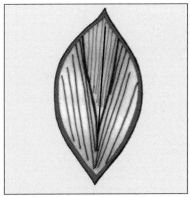

Fig 18.23 Blunt dissection of the sternohyoid muscle

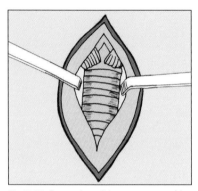

Fig 18.24 Retraction of the sternomastoid and sternohyoid muscles

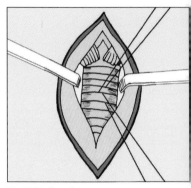

Fig 18.25 Attach stay sutures

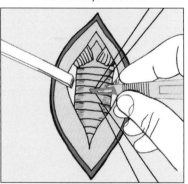

Fig 18.26 Tracheotomy

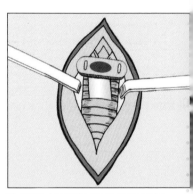

Fig 18.27 Insert the tracheotomy tube (towards lung)

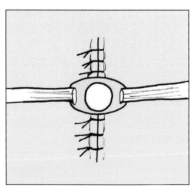

Fig 18.28 Fixate the tracheotomy tube/skin suture

Method

- **Preparation**
  - Sedation (no sedation in case of acute laryngeal obstruction)
  - Dorsal position
  - Clip the fur/disinfect the skin

- **Technique**
  - Make a longitudinal skin incision over the trachea
  - Perform a blunt dissection of the sternohyoid muscle
  - Place the retractors (BEWARE of the thyroid)
  - Make a transverse incision between the second–third or third–fourth tracheal ring
  - Insert the tracheal tube towards the lung
  - Close the wound
  - Fixate the tracheal tube (skin sutures or tie)

- **Care/maintenance**
  - Humidify the air
  - Remove the secretion/suction every 2–4 hours
  - Clean with saline

Complications

- Damage to the thyroid
- Damage to the vocal chords
- Local infection
- Pneumonia
- Obstruction of the tube
- Subcutaneous emphysema

Inhalation Therapy

Indication

- Inhalation of medication via the breathing air (antibiotics, antimycotics, acetylcysteine)
- Bronchopneumonia

Inhalation Therapy

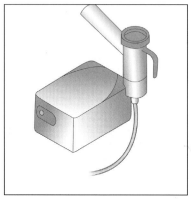

Fig 18.29 Parey-Boy®-Inhalator

Method

- **Preparation**
  - Oxygen tent/modified Elizabethan collar, cage or transport box covered with cling film
  - Inhalator: Parey-Boy®

- **Technique**
  - dilute medications with water/saline

19 Parenteral Nutrition

Pharyngostomy Tube

Indication

- Inappetence/dysphagia (difficulty in swallowing/chewing)

Pharyngostomy Tube

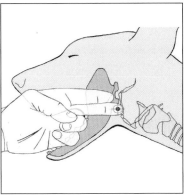

Fig 19.1 Palpation of the puncture site

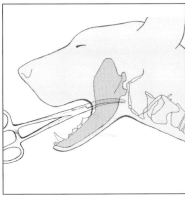

Fig 19.2 Insertion of a pair of curved artery forceps

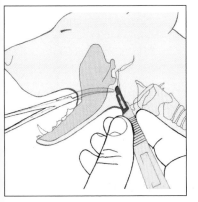

Fig 19.3 Skin incision over the tip of the artery forceps

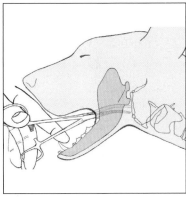

Fig 19.4 Advance the artery forceps through the opening

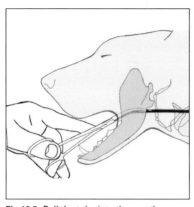

Fig 19.5 Pull the tube into the mouth

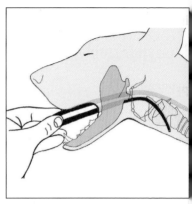

Fig 19.6 Push the tube into the oesophagus and stomach

Method

- **Preparation**
  - Sedation
  - Possibly endotracheal intubation

- **Technique**
  - Palpate the puncture site through the mouth (hyoid bone and mandible)
  - Consider marking the puncture site on the skin
  - Feed a curved artery forceps through the mouth to the puncture site
  - Palpate the puncture site over the tip of the artery forceps
  - Make an incision over the tip of the artery forceps
  - Advance the artery forceps until it is visible through the incision
  - Open the artery forceps and grasp the tube with it
  - Pull the tube with the artery forceps through the mouth
  - Push the tip of the tube manually into the oesophagus and stomach
  - Fixate the tube with adhesive tape and a skin suture
  - Place a bandage and Elizabethan collar

- **Care/maintenance**
  - Flush the tube before and after each application of nutritional fluid with saline
  - Daily dressing change

Complications

- Haemorrhages
- Infection

Percutaneous Endoscopic Gastrostomy (PEG Tube)

Indication

- Dysphagia
- Oesophageal obstruction

PEG Tube

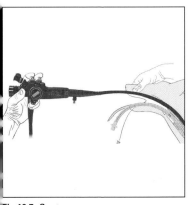

Fig 19.7 Gastroscopy

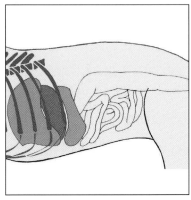

Fig 19.8 Physiological position of the stomach

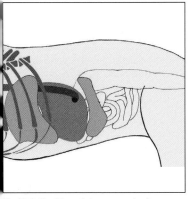

Fig 19.9 Position of the stomach after inflation with air

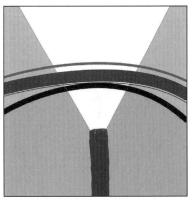

Fig 19.10 Localisation of the puncture site

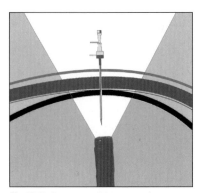

Fig 19.11 Puncture of the stomach

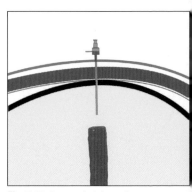

Fig 19.12 Removal of the stylet

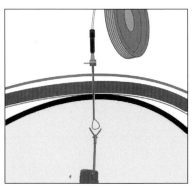

Fig 19.13 Feed the double thread through the catheter

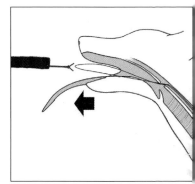

Fig 19.14 Pull the double thread through the mouth

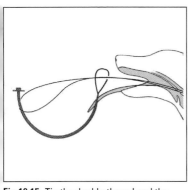

Fig 19.15 Tie the double thread and the PEG tube together

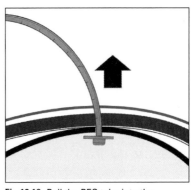

Fig 19.16 Pull the PEG tube into the stomach

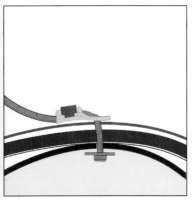

Fig 19.17 Fixation of the PEG tube with the external bumper

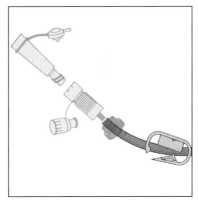

Fig 19.18 Attachments and tubing clamp

Method

- **System**
  - Freka® PEG Set Gastral CH/FR 15, Fresenius Kabi

- **Preparation**
  - Sedation
  - Possibly endotracheal intubation

- **Technique**
  - Gastroscopy

- Inflate the stomach with air
- Localise the puncture site on the left abdominal wall caudal of the ribs (light beam of the gastroscope is visible through the abdominal wall)
- Puncture the stomach above the light source with the puncture cannula and plastic catheter
- Remove the stylet
- Attach a guiding aid and feed the double thread through the catheter, until it is visible through the endoscope
- Draw back the guiding aid (air valve seal)
- Insert the biopsy forceps into the biopsy channel of the endoscope
- Grab the double thread with the biopsy forceps
- Pull the double thread and the endoscope out through the mouth
- Tie the double thread together with the PEG tube
- Pull the PEG tube into the stomach by pulling slowly on the other end of the double thread
- Pull the PEG tube and the plastic catheter through the abdominal wall, until the internal bumper lies flat against the stomach wall
- Cut the double thread at the base of the tube
- Fixate the PEG tube with the external bumper
- Attach the tubing clamp
- Cut off the end of the PEG tube
- Place attachments
- Apply a dressing
- Use an Elizabethan collar

- **Care/maintenance**
    - Flush the tube before and after each application of nutritional fluid with saline
    - Daily dressing change
    - Rotate and shift the tube daily

Complications

- Pressure necrosis (stomach)
- Infection
- Peritonitis
- Ingrowth of the tube
- Vomitus

Nasogastric Tube

Indication

- Dysphagia without obstruction

Nasogastric Tube

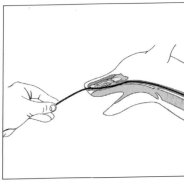

Fig 19.19 Insert the gastric tube through the nose

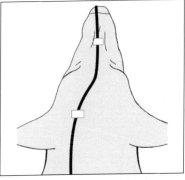

Fig 19.20 Fixate the nasogastric tube

Method

- **Preparation**
  - Possibly slight sedation
  - Standing/sternal or prone position

- **Technique**
  - Apply a lidocaine solution intranasally
  - Moisten the nasogastric tube with lidocaine gel
  - Insert the nasogastric tube slowly into the stomach while the head is slightly flexed
  - Palpate the larynx in order to stimulate swallowing
  - Check the correct position of the tube inside the stomach: visual control through the mouth
  - Instil 2ml of saline (this causes a cough in case of an intratracheal placement)
  - Fixate the nasogastric tube via adhesive tape and skin suture
  - Use an Elizabethan collar
  - Check the correct position with an X-ray

- **Care/maintenance**
  - Flush the tube before and after each application of nutritional fluid with saline

20 Urinary Catheter

Urethral Catheter

Indication

- Urine drainage in case of urinary retention/overflow bladder
- Placeholder during penis amputation, perineal hernia operations

Urinary catheter in the male dog

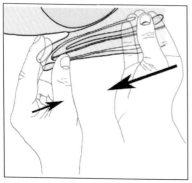

Fig 20.1 Extrude the penis

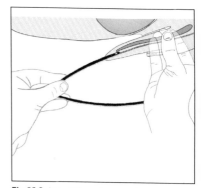

Fig 20.2 Insert the urinary catheter

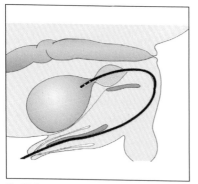

Fig 20.3 Position of the urinary catheter

Method

- **Preparation**
  - Standing/lateral recumbency/dorsal position
  - Extrude the penis
  - Clean the penis in case of balanoposthitis
  - Measure the length of the urinary catheter (sterile gloves)
  - Apply sterile lubrication/saline onto the tip of the urinary catheter

- **Technique**
  - Fixate the penis onto the penile bone
  - Insert the urinary catheter into the urethra (sterility) until it reaches the bladder neck
  - Catch the urine in a sterile tube
  - Remove the urinary catheter

Complications

- Knotting of the urinary catheter inside the urinary bladder
- Infection
- Perforation of the urethra/bladder

Urinary Catheter in the Male Cat

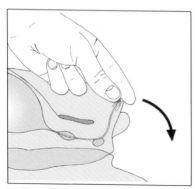

Fig 20.4 Extrude and horizontalise the penis

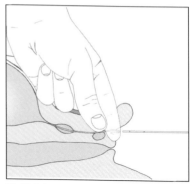

Fig 20.5 Insert the urinary catheter

Method

- **Preparation**
  - Sedation
  - Dorsal position
  - Extrude and horizontalise the penis
  - Apply some sterile lubrication gel/saline onto the tip of the urinary catheter

- **Technique**
  - Fixate the penis at the prepuce
  - Insert the urinary catheter into the urethra (sterility) until it reaches the bladder neck, possibly while slightly twisting it
  - Catch the urine in a sterile tube
  - Remove the urinary catheter (possibly fixate it via skin suture in case of urinary obstruction)

Complications

- Perforation of urethra/urinary bladder
- Infection

Urinary catheter in the female dog and cat: flexible catheter

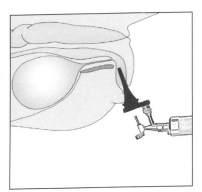

Fig 20.6 Insert the otoscope/speculum vertically

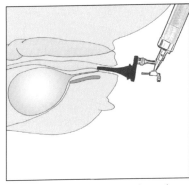

Fig 20.7 Advance the otoscope/speculum horizontally

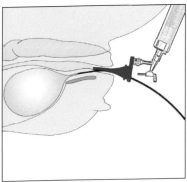

Fig 20.8 Insert the urinary catheter under visual control

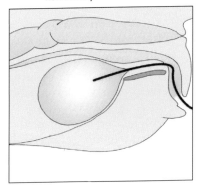

Fig 20.9 Position of the urinary catheter

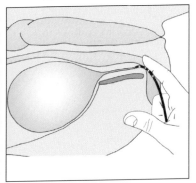

Fig 20.10 Insert the urinary catheter under digital control

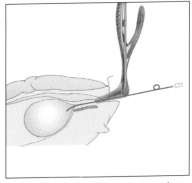

Fig 20.11 Insert the metal catheter under visual control

Method

- **Preparation**
  - Standing
  - Part the vulvar labia
  - Apply some sterile lubrication gel/saline onto the tip of the urinary catheter

- **Technique**

  Flexible catheter (under visual control)
  - Measure the length of the urinary catheter
  - Insert the otoscope/speculum vertically into the vulva while avoiding the clitoris (lift the speculum a little)
  - Advance the otoscope/speculum horizontally until the urethral opening is reached (ventral)
  - Insert the urinary catheter under visual control
  - Advance the urinary catheter
  - Catch the urine in a sterile tube
  - Remove the urinary catheter and the otoscope/speculum

  Flexible catheter (under digital control)
  - Measure the length of the urinary catheter
  - Insert urinary catheter vertically into the vulva using fingers while avoiding the clitoris
  - Advance horizontally until the urethral opening is reached
  - Insert the urinary catheter digitally into the urethra
  - Advance the urinary catheter
  - Catch the urine in a sterile tube
  - Remove the urinary catheter

  Metal catheter (under visual control)
  - Insert the speculum vertically into the vulva while avoiding the clitoris (lift the speculum a little)
  - Advance the speculum horizontally until the urethral opening is reached (ventral)
  - Spread the speculum
  - Insert the urinary catheter under visual control
  - Advance the urinary catheter
  - Catch the urine in a sterile tube
  - Remove the urinary catheter and the speculum

Complications

- Perforation of the urethra/bladder
- Infection

Pre-Pubic Urinary Catheter

Indication

- Urine drainage in neurogenic micturition disorders

Pre-Pubic Urinary Catheter

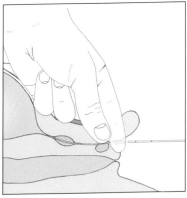

Fig 20.12 Urinary catheterisation

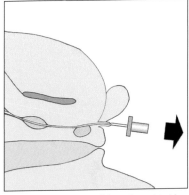

Fig 20.13 Evacuation of the urinary bladder

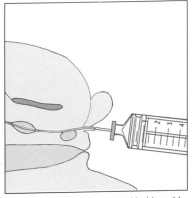

Fig 20.14 Filling of the urinary bladder with physiological saline

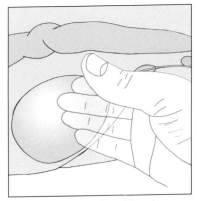

Fig 20.15 Manual fixation of the urinary bladder

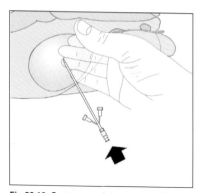

Fig 20.16 Cystocentesis/catheter with a splittable cannula

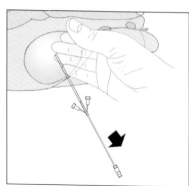

Fig 20.17 Removal of the stylet

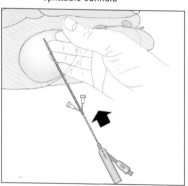

Fig 20.18 Insert the Foley catheter into the cannula

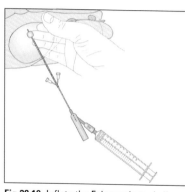

Fig 20.19 Inflate the Foley catheter balloon

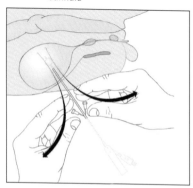

Fig 20.20 Divide and remove the catheter

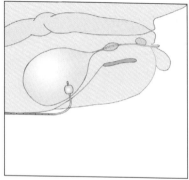

Fig 20.21 Fixation on the skin/bandage

Method

- **Preparation**
  - Sedation
  - Dorsal position/lateral recumbency
  - Clip the fur/disinfect the skin
  - Catheterize and fill the urinary bladder with physiological saline

- **Technique**
  - Fixate the urinary bladder manually
  - Make a stab incision of the skin paramedian over the puncture site
  - Puncture the urinary bladder with a catheter containing a splittable cannula (Splittocan®, Peel-Away® Catheter)
  - Insert a Foley catheter through the cannula (Foley catheter 5F, 12 inch)
  - Inflate the Foley catheter balloon with physiological saline
  - Evacuate the urinary bladder
  - Pull the Foley catheter back to the abdominal wall
  - Check the correct position via X-rays or ultrasound
  - Fixate the catheter to the skin with exiting of the catheter caudal of the shoulder)
  - Apply a bandage with antibiotic cream/Elizabethan collar

Care/maintenance
  - Evacuate the urinary bladder 3–4 times daily
  - Instil 5ml of lavasept® solution 0.05 per cent after the bladder has been emptied
  - Bandage change

Complications

- Infection (cystitis/peritonitis)
- Uroabdomen
- Necrosis of the bladder wall
- Patient may pull out the catheter

21 Drainage

Thoracocentesis/Thoracic Drainage

Indication

- Relief of a thoracic effusion
- Relief of a tension pneumothorax

Thoracocentesis

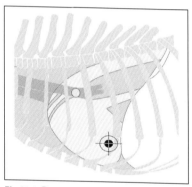

Fig 21.1 Puncture site for the drainage of a thoracic effusion

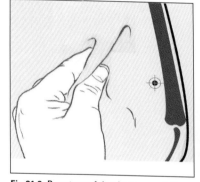

Fig 21.2 Puncture of the thorax cranial to the rib

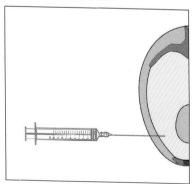

Fig 21.3 Puncture of the thorax with a needle and syringe

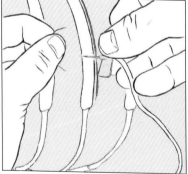

Fig 21.4 Puncture of the thorax with a butterfly catheter

Method

- **Preparation**
  - While the patient is standing on the examination table clip the fur and disinfect the skin (left/right thoracic wall)
  - System: 10ml syringe with three-way tap and an attached cannula or butterfly catheter (cat)

- **Technique**
  - Puncture site: cranial of the rib in the seventh–eighth intercostal space, dorsal (if pneumothorax), ventral (if pleural effusion)
  - Push the skin to cranial
  - Puncture the thoracic wall slowly
  - Aspirate air/fluid until a negative pressure has been created
  - Possibly close the three-way tap, change the syringe, open the three-way tap again and repeat aspiration
  - Remove the puncture needle while maintaining the insertion angle
  - Let go of the skin that was previously moved forward
  - Compress the puncture site (2–5 min)
  - Examine/process the sample
  - Take control radiographs

Complications

- Thoracic haemorrhage (rib vessels, lung puncture)
- Pneumothorax (lung puncture, leak)
- Subcutaneous emphysema
- Infection

Thoracic Drainage

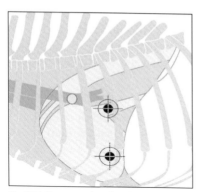

Fig 21.5 Puncture sites for air and effusive drainage

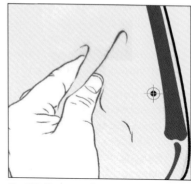

Fig 21.6 Puncture of the thorax cranial to the rib

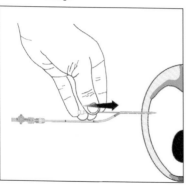

Fig 21.7 Puncture of the thorax

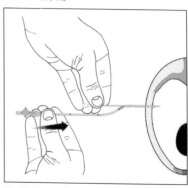

Fig 21.8 Insertion of the thoracic drain over the trocar

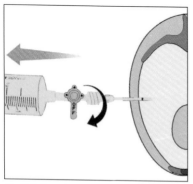

Fig 21.9 Attachment of the syringe and opening of the two-way tap

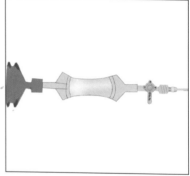

Fig 21.10 Thoracic drain with a valve and gaiter

Method

- **Preparation**
  - While the patient is standing on the examination table
  - Clip the fur and disinfect the skin
  - Subcutaneous topical anaesthesia
  - System: drain (8,5 FR), two-way tap, trocar (Global Veterinary Prod.)

- **Technique**
  - Puncture site: cranial of the rib in the seventh–eighth intercostal space, dorsal (in case of pneumothorax), ventral (in case of thoracic effusion)
  - Push the skin towards cranial
  - Close the two-way tap
  - Puncture the thorax
  - Insert the drain towards cranial over the trocar
  - Remove the trocar
  - Fixate the drain to the skin
  - Drain the fluid/air (suction pump/syringe)
  - In case of pneumothorax: attach a valve (Heimlich valve/Leo valve) and gaiter
  - Take control radiographs
  - Thoracic bandage

Complications

- Thoracic haemorrhage (rib vessels, lung puncture)
- Pneumothorax (lung puncture, leak)
- Subcutaneous emphysema
- Infection

Pericardiocentesis/Pericardial Drainage

Indication

- Relief of a pericardial effusion

Pericardiocentesis

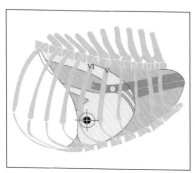

Fig 21.11 Puncture site

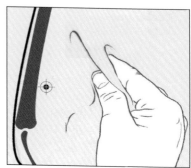

Fig 21.12 Puncture of the thorax cranial to the rib

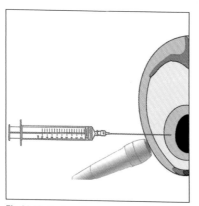

Fig 21.13 Pericardial puncture with a needle and syringe

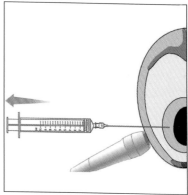

Fig 21.14 Aspiration

Method

- **Preparation**
  - Position: left lateral recumbency, sternal, possibly standing
  - Clip the fur and disinfect the skin
  - System: venous catheter, three-way tap, syringe
  - ECG-control
  - Ultrasound-control

- **Technique**
  - Push the skin over the puncture site towards cranial
  - Pericardial puncture: right thoracic wall, in the fifth intercostal space, cranial of the rib near the chondrocostal junction, puncture horizontally while lightly aspirating
  - Drainage
  - Change the syringe after closing the three-way tap
  - Remove the puncture cannula and compress the puncture site
  - Check if the aspirate is coagulating: no coagulation in case of a pericardial effusion, coagulation in case of a cardiac puncture
  - Take control radiographs

Complications

- Haemorrhage
- Pneumothorax
- Ventricular ectopic complexes
- Heart perforation
- Lung perforation
- Infection
- Recurrence

Pericardial Drainage (Venous catheter)

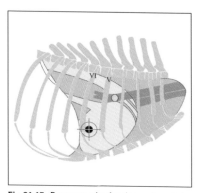

Fig 21.15 Puncture site for the pericardial drainage

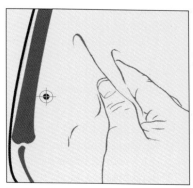

Fig 21.16 Puncture cranial of the rib

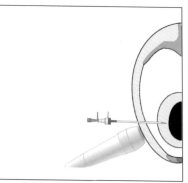

Fig 21.17 Pericardial puncture with a venous catheter

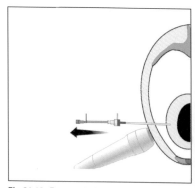

Fig 21.18 Removal of the stylet

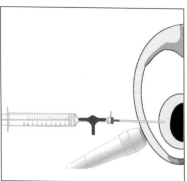

Fig 21.19 Attachment of the three-way tap/syringe and aspiration

Method

- **Preparation**
  - Position: left lateral recumbency, sternal, possibly standing
  - Clip the fur and disinfect the skin
  - System: venous catheter, three-way tap, syringe
  - ECG-control
  - Ultrasound-control

- **Technique**
  - Push the skin over the puncture site towards cranial
  - Perform a pericardial puncture with the venous catheter system
  - Right thoracic wall, fifth intercostal space, cranial of the rib near the chondrocostal junction
  - Puncture horizontally, until the fluid flows into the catheter
  - Remove the stylet while fixating the catheter
  - Attach the syringe with the three-way tap/apply suction
  - Drain
  - Change the syringe after closing the three-way tap
  - Remove the puncture cannula and compress the puncture site
  - Check if the aspirate is coagulating: no coagulation in case of a pericardial effusion, coagulation in case of a cardiac puncture
  - Take control radiographs

Complications

- Haemorrhage
- Pneumothorax
- Ventricular ectopic complexes
- Heart perforation
- Lung perforation
- Infection
- Recurrence

Pericardial Drainage (Pigtail catheter)

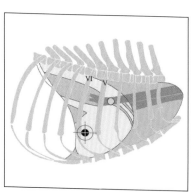

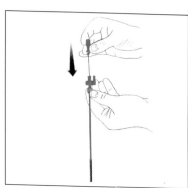

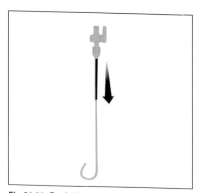

Fig 21.20 Push the straightener forwards

Fig 21.21 Insert the steel stylet

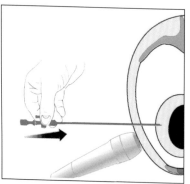

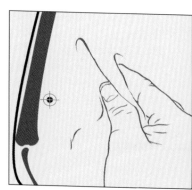

Fig 21.22 Puncture site

Fig 21.23 Puncture cranial of the rib

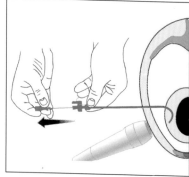

Fig 21.24 Pericardial puncture (cross section)

Fig 21.25 Push the pigtail catheter forwards

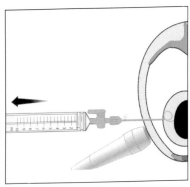

Fig 21.26 Attach a syringe and aspirate

Method

- **Preparation**
  - Positioning: left lateral recumbency, sternal or prone position, possibly standing
  - Clip the fur, disinfect the skin
  - System: Pigtail catheter with a two-way tap, syringe
  - ECG control
  - Ultrasound control
  - Pigtail catheter: push the straightener forwards and insert the steel stylet

- **Technique**
  - Push the skin over the puncture site towards cranial
  - Perform a pericardial puncture with the pigtail catheter system (two-way tap open)
  - Right thoracic wall, fifth intercostal space, cranial of the rib near the chondrocostal junction
  - puncture horizontally, until the fluid flows into the catheter
  - Remove the stylet while fixating the catheter
  - Close the two-way tap
  - Advance the pigtail catheter
  - Attach a syringe with a two-way tap/suction and drainage
  - Take control radiographs

Complications

- Haemorrhage
- Perforation of the heart
- Ventricular extrasystole
- Pneumothorax
- Perforation of the lung
- Infection

Abdominocentesis/Abdominal Drainage

Indication

- Relief of an abdominal effusion

Abdominocentesis

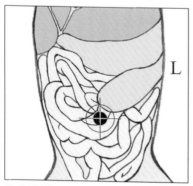

Fig 21.27 Puncture site for abdominocentesis

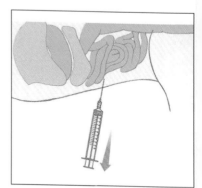

Fig 21.28 Abdominal puncture with a syringe/needle and aspiration

Method

- **Preparation**
  - Lateral recumbency
  - Clip the fur and disinfect the skin

- **Technique**
  - Possibly evacuation of urinary bladder required
  - Puncture the abdominal wall paramedian and caudal of the umbilicus (use a syringe with an attached hypodermic needle)
  - Direct the puncture needle towards caudal
  - Aspirate
  - Remove the syringe and needle

Complications

- Splenic puncture
- Intestinal puncture
- Puncture of the urinary bladder
- Peritonitis

Abdominal Drainage/Peritoneal Drainage

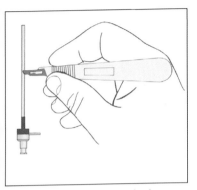

Fig 21.29 Cutting holes into a plastic venous catheter

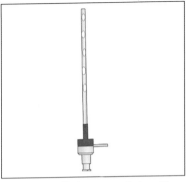

Fig 21.30 Modified venous catheter with holes

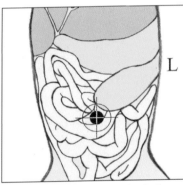

Fig 21.31 Puncture site for abdominal drainage

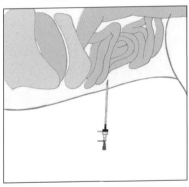

Fig 21.32 Abdominal puncture with a venous catheter

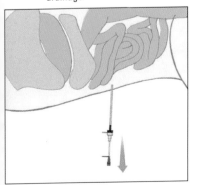

Fig 21.33 Removal of the steel stylet

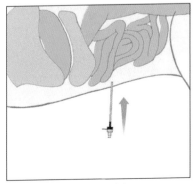

Fig 21.34 Advancement of the venous catheter

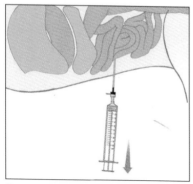

Fig 21.35 Attachment of the syringe and aspiration

Method

- **Preparation**
  - Lateral recumbency
  - Clip the fur/disinfect the skin

- **Technique**
  - Cut holes into a large venous catheter
  - Possibly empty the bladder
  - Puncture the abdominal wall carefully paramedian and caudal to the umbilicus
  - Direct the puncture needle towards caudal
  - Withdraw the steel stylet
  - Advance the plastic catheter
  - Remove the steel stylet
  - Insert the plastic catheter
  - Attach the syringe
  - Aspirate

Complications

- Blockage of the catheter/rearrangement by the greater omentum
- Intestinal puncture
- Puncture of the urinary bladder

Paracentesis

Indication

- Relief of a middle ear effusion by puncture of the tympanic membrane

Paracentesis/Myringotomy

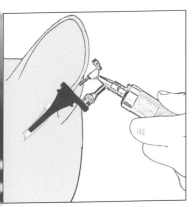

Fig 21.36 Otoscopic examination

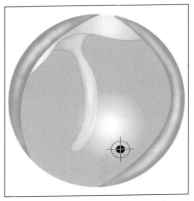

Fig 21.37 Puncture site of the tympanic membrane for paracentesis

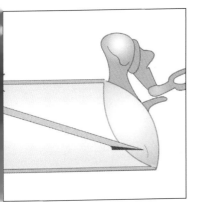

Fig 21.38 Paracentesis with a paracentesis knife

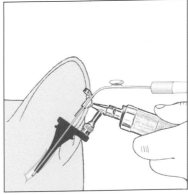

Fig 21.39 Suction of the secretion in the external ear canal/in front of the tympanic membrane

Method

- **Preparation**
  - Sternal/prone position

- **Technique**
  - Otoscopic examination
  - X–ray examination (tympanic bulla)
  - Clean the external ear canal
  - Puncture the tympanic membrane with a paracentesis knife in the lower right quadrant
  - Suction the secretion off in the external ear canal outside the tympanic membrane
  - Insert 4–5 drops of ciprofloxacin/enrofloxacin injection solution into the external ear canal

Complications

- Damage to the auditory ossicles while puncturing the tympanic membrane
- Accidental suction of the auditory ossicles

22 Flushes

Nasal Flush

Indication

- Obstructive rhinitis
- Foreign bodies beyond the reach for the endoscope

Retrograde Nasal Flush

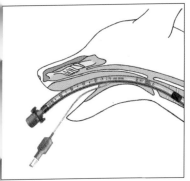

Fig 22.1 Endotracheal intubation

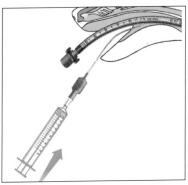

Fig 22.2 Cuffing of the endotracheal tube

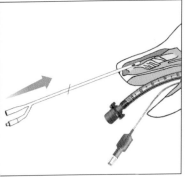

Fig 22.3 Endonasal insertion of a Foley catheter

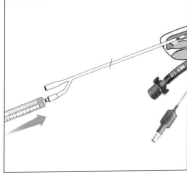

Fig 22.4 Inflation of the balloon of the Foley catheter

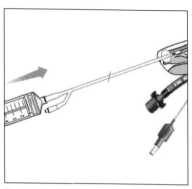

Fig 22.5 Retrograde nasal flush

Method

- **Preparation**
  - General anaesthesia
  - Lateral recumbency with lowered head position
  - Endotracheal intubation with cuffing of the tube

- **Technique**
  - Insertion of a Foley catheter (5F) endonasally for 1–2cm into the dorsal nasal passage
  - Inflate the balloon of the Foley catheter with physiological saline
  - Flush with bodywarm saline while ensuring the patient is breathing and the fluid discharges through the oral cavity

Complications

- Aspiration of fluid

Orthograde Nasal Flush

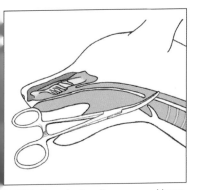

Fig 22.6 Curved artery forceps as guidance aid

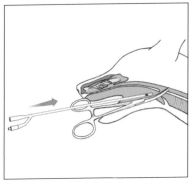

Fig 22.7 Insertion of the Foley catheter through the mouth

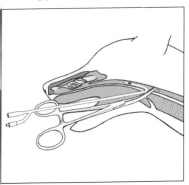

Fig 22.8 Insertion of the Foley catheter into the nasopharynx

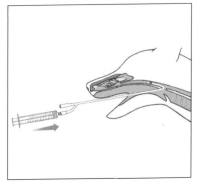

Fig 22.9 Inflation of the balloon of the Foley catheter

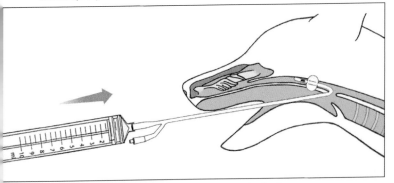

Fig 22.10 Orthograde nasal flush with bodywarm physiological saline

Method

- **Preparation**
  - General anaesthesia
  - Lateral recumbency with lowered head position
  - In combination with retrograde nasal flush in order to instil antimycotics in case of aspergillosis

- **Technique**
  - Insert a Foley catheter (5F) for 1–2cm into the nasopharynx with the assistance of curved artery forceps
  - Inflate the balloon of the Foley catheter with physiological saline
  - Flush with bodywarm saline while checking the pharynx

Complications

- Incomplete inflation of the balloon of the Foley catheter and aspiration of fluid

Nasolacrimal Duct Flush

Indication

- Obstruction

Nasolacrimal Duct Flush

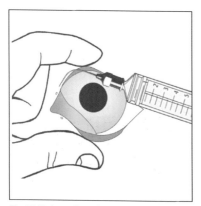

Fig 22.11 Insertion of the cannula into the upper lacrimal opening

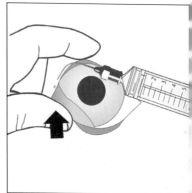

Fig 22.12 Hold the lower lacrimal duct opening closed and flush

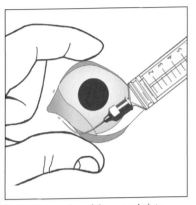

Fig 22.13 Insertion of the cannula into lower lacrimal duct opening

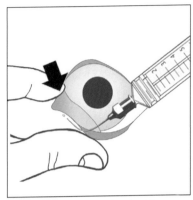

Fig 22.14 Hold the upper lacrimal duct opening closed and flush

Method

- **Preparation**
  - Sternal/prone position
  - Sedation
  - Fluorescein test

- **Technique**
  - Hold the eyelids open with one hand
  - Insert the flushing cannula with an attached syringe from lateral into the lacrimal duct
  - Compress the other lacrimal duct opening of the same eye with your fingers
  - Flush with bodywam physiological saline

Complications

- Rupture of the nasolacrimal duct in case of stenosis

Ear Flush

Indication

- Cleaning of the ears prior to commencement of treatment

Ear Cleaning/Ear Flush

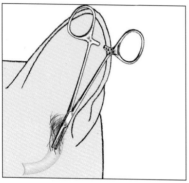

Fig 22.15 Possibly removal of hair from the external ear canal

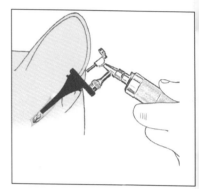

Fig 22.16 Otoscopic examination

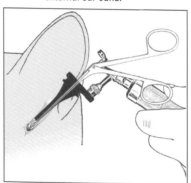

Fig 22.17 Possibly removal of a foreign body (awn/grass seed)

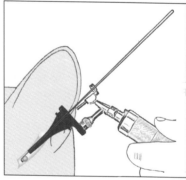

Fig 22.18 Possibly removal of a plug with a hook

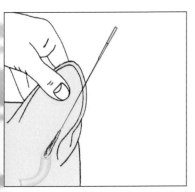

Fig 22.19 Removal of wax with a cotton bud

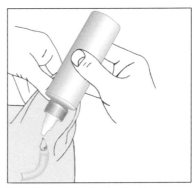

Fig 22.20 Instil the flushing liquid

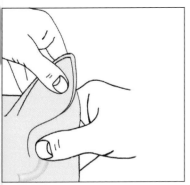

Fig 22.21 Massage flushing liquid in well

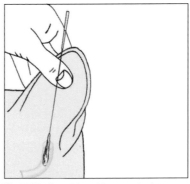

Fig 22.22 Clean/dry with cotton buds

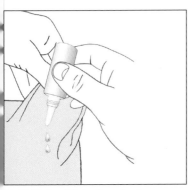

Fig 22.23 Possibly instil medication

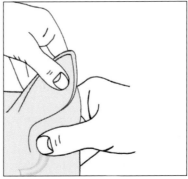

Fig 22.24 Massage medication in well

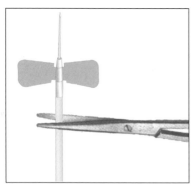

Fig 22.25 Modified flushing catheter made from a butterfly catheter

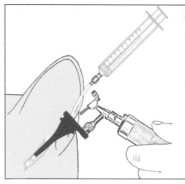

Fig 22.26 Flush and suction while maintaining visual control

Method

- **Preparation**
  - Ear cleaning: no sedation, ear flush: sedation

- **Technique**
  - Ear cleaning/ear flushing
  - Remove some hair from the external ear canal if required (poodle)
  - Otoscopic examination (contraindication for ear flush: rupture of the tympanic membrane)
  - Remove a plug or foreign body from the ear if present
  - Instil commercial ear cleaning solution into the external ear canal (until it flows over)
  - Massage the external ear canal
  - Clean and dry the external ear canal with cotton buds and cotton wool
  - Allow the patient to shake their head
  - Clean and dry the external ear canal with a cotton bud and cotton wool
  - Instil medication into the external ear canal if required
  - Massage the external ear canal

Ear cleaning with a flushing catheter

  - Modify/cut a flushing catheter from a butterfly catheter
  - Attach a syringe
  - Insert the flushing catheter into the otoscope funnel
  - Flush the ears and suction off the flushing liquid

Complications

- Rupture of the tympanic membrane
- Otitis media/vestibular syndrome in case of a ruptured tympanic membrane

Peritoneal Lavage

Indication

- Peritonitis
- Acotaemia in renal failure

Peritoneal Lavage

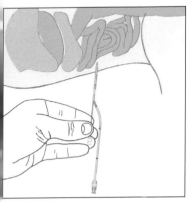

Fig 22.27 Puncture of the abdomen

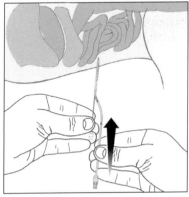

Fig 22.28 Removal of the trocar

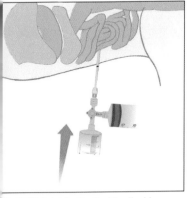

Fig 22.29 Inlet for the flushing liquid

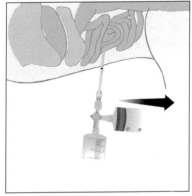

Fig 22.30 Outlet for the flushing liquid

Method

- **System**
  - 8.5 French Trocar Catheter, Global® Veterinary Products

- **Preparation**
  - Lateral recumbency
  - Clip the fur/disinfect the skin
  - Topical anaesthesia
  - Possibly evacuation of the bladder

- **Technique**
  - Puncture the abdominal wall paramedian and caudal to the umbilicus
  - Direct the puncture needle towards caudal
  - Insert the catheter with help of the trocar
  - Remove the trocar
  - Attach a three-way tap
  - Attach and label a 50ml syringe to the inlet and outlet of the flushing port
  - Fixate the catheter to the skin
  - Instil bodywam flushing liquid at a dose of 20ml/kg (e.g., 1 l Ringerlactate solution + 30ml Glucose 50 per cent solution)
  - Drain after about 30 min
  - Repeat the procedure after 2 hours
  - Apply a bandage
  - Use an Elizabethan collar

Complications

- Blockage of the catheter/rearrangement by the greater omentum
- Intestinal puncture
- Puncture of the urinary bladder
- Peritonitis

Gastric Lavage

Indication

- Poisoning
- Gastric dilation/volvulus

Gastric Lavage

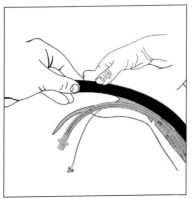

Fig 22.31 Insertion of a wide gastric tube

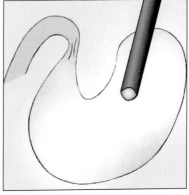

Fig 22.32 Gastric tube inside the stomach

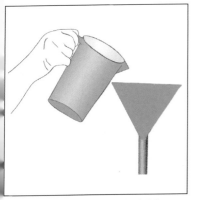

Fig 22.33 Attach a funnel and administer the flushing liquid

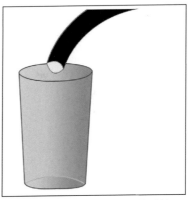

Fig 22.34 Outflow of the flushing liquid into a bucket

Method

- **Preparation**
  - Sedation
  - Endotracheal intubation with cuffing of the tube
  - Dorsal position
- **Technique**
  - Insert the gastric tube into the stomach (garden or industrial hose with the widest possible diameter)
  - Check the correct position of the gastric tube inside the stomach (via auscultation/palpation)
  - Hold the gastric tube up
  - Attach a funnel
  - Instil bodywarm flushing liquid (tap water)
  - Let the flushing liquid run out into the bucket on the floor
  - Repeat the procedure until the flushing liquid looks clear
  - Bend and remove the gastric tube

Complications

- Aspiration
- Perforation of the stomach/oesophagus

Colonic Lavage

Indication

- Constipation/coprostasis

Colonic Lavage

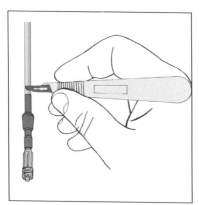

Fig 22.35 Modified flushing catheter made from an infusion line

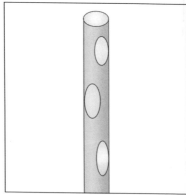

Fig 22.36 Flushing catheter with holes

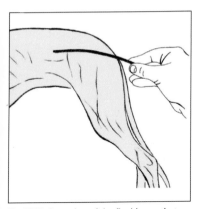

Fig 22.37 Insertion of the flushing catheter into the rectum

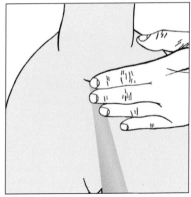

Fig 22.38 Hold the anus closed

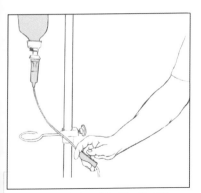

Fig 22.39 Instillation of flushing liquid for the cat (physiological saline)

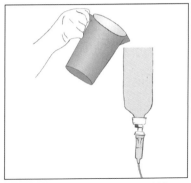

Fig 22.40 Instillation of flushing liquid for the dog (tap water)

Method

- **Preparation**
  - Sedation
  - Modify an infusion line by cutting end and side openings into it
  - Moisten the flushing catheter and anus with lubricant/paraffin
- **Technique**
  - Insert the modified flushing tube into the rectum while applying manual control
  - Hold the anus closed with your hand
  - Infuse the flushing liquid into the rectum: bodywarm physiological saline in cats, bodywarm tap water in dogs
  - Massage the colon manually from abdominal
  - Remove the hand that is holding the anus shut and let the flushing liquid run out
  - Repeat the procedure until all faeces have been removed from the descending colon
  - Remove the flushing tube

Complications

- Haemorrhages
- Perforation of the colon
- Anaemia (cat)
- Hypothermia
- Vomitus
- Faecal incontinence
- Megacolon

Anal Sac Lavage

Indication

- Impaction/anal sac abscess

Anal Sac Lavage

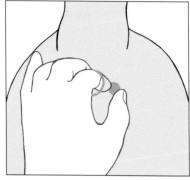

Fig 22.41 Internal expression of the anal sacs

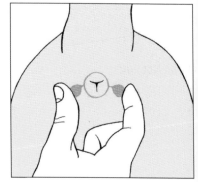

Fig 22.42 External expression of the anal sacs

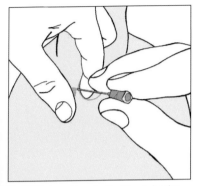

Fig 22.43 Insertion of a flushing/irrigation cannula

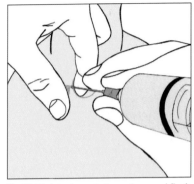

Fig 22.44 Attachment of a syringe and flush

Method

- **Preparation**
  - The patient is standing on the examination table
  - Moisten the anus with lubricant/paraffin
  - Express the anal sac internally

- **Technique**
  - Probe the anal sac with a blunt curved lacrimal duct or irrigation cannula
  - Attach a syringe containing the flushing liquid (usually povidone iodine solution)
  - Flush the anal sac
  - Express the anal sac internally
  - Apply medication into the anal sac (usually an antibiotic)

Complications

- Damage to the excretory duct
- Perforation of the anal sac
- Painfulness

Urethral Lavage

Indication

- Obstruction of the urinary tract/urolithiasis

Urethral lavage in the male cat

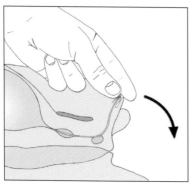

Fig 22.45 Extrusion and horizontalisation of the penis

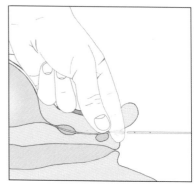

Fig 22.46 Insertion of a urinary catheter up to the obstruction

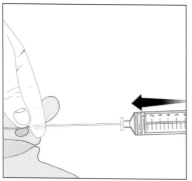

Fig 22.47 Urethral lavage

Method

- **Preparation**
  - Intravenous catheter
  - Infusion therapy according to the potassium level (usually physiological saline)
  - Sedation (usually avoidance of ketamine)
  - Dorsal position
  - Cystocentesis for pressure release
  - Extrusion and horizontalisation of the penis
  - Application of sterile lubricant/saline onto the tip of the urinary catheter

- **Technique**
  - Fixate the penis at the prepuce
  - Insert the urinary catheter into the urethra under sterile conditions until the obstruction is reached, possibly while rotating it slightly
  - Perform a urethral lavage with bodywarm physiological saline (5ml syringe)
  - Insert the urinary catheter into the bladder while flushing
  - Fixate the urinary catheter on the skin

Complications

- Perforation of the urethra
- Initial hyperkalaemia, in post-obstructive polyuric phase, hypokalaemia

Urethral lavage in the male dog: urohydropulsion

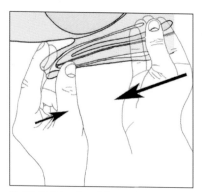

Fig 22.48 Extrusion of the penis

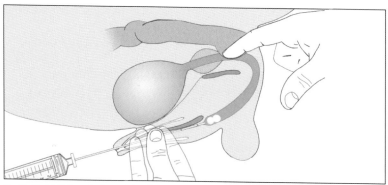

Fig 22.49 Digital occlusion of the distal urethra

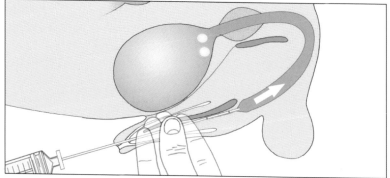

Fig 22.50 Digital occlusion of the urethral opening

Method

- **Preparation**
  - Intravenous catheter
  - Infusion therapy according to the potassium level (usually physiological saline)
  - Possibly sedation (usually avoidance of ketamine)
  - Dorsal position or lateral recumbency
  - Possibly cystocentesis for pressure release
  - Extrusion of the penis
  - Apply sterile lubricant/physiological saline onto the tip of the urinary catheter

- **Technique**
  - Fixate the penis on the penis bone
  - Insert the urinary catheter into the urethra until the obstruction is reached (uroliths)
  - Occlude the distal urethra via rectal digital pressure
  - Flush with physiolical saline (10ml syringe) for urethral dilation
  - Release the digital pressure
  - Flush while occluding the urethral opening

Complications

- Perforation of the urethra or urinary bladder
- Infection
- Hyperkalaemia/hypokalaemia

23 Bandages

Ruff

Indication

- Licking of wounds
- Self-mutilation

Elizabethan Collar

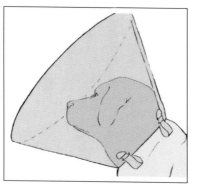

Fig 23.1 Elizabethan collar/pet cone

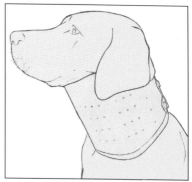

Fig 23.2 Neck brace

Method

- **Technique**
  - Choose the appropriate size: it should reach a few cm beyond the tip of the nose
  - Assemble the collar according to the model instructions (usual strap guide out-in-out)
  - Attach to the dog's usual collar or a doubled gauze strip for the cat
  - Leave a space of two fingers width between the collar and the ventral neck

Complications

- Panic
- Impaired movement
- Inappetence
- Collar slips off
- Catching of limbs inside the cone (cat)
- Local skin irritation

Spray/Plaster/Stulpa Dressing

Indication

- Protective dressing after surgical procedures

Spray/Plaster/Stulpa Dressing

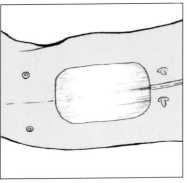

Fig 23.3 Plaster

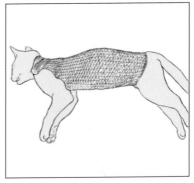

Fig 23.4 Stulpa dressing

Method

- **Technique**

  Spray dressing
  - Aluminium spray, methylenblue spray
  - Plaster
  - Clip the fur
  - Clean and disinfect the wound
  - Apply surgical adhesive spray around the edges of the plaster if required
  - Cut to use (rounding of the edges as necessary) and apply the plaster

  Stulpa Dressing
  - Choose the appropriate size
  - Cut to use (openings for the forelimbs)
  - Put on the dressing (from cranial to caudal)
  - Fixate the dressing (knotting over the gluteal region)

Complications

- Skin irritation

Ear Dressing

Indication

- Protective dressing after surgical procedures

Wound Dressing

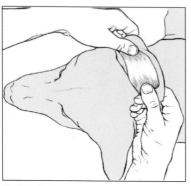

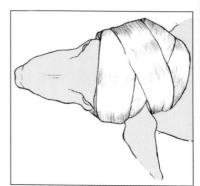

Fig 23.5 Unilateral ear dressing (step 1)

Fig 23.6 Unilateral ear dressing (step 2)

Method

- **Technique**
  - Fold the affected ear over the top of the head
  - Possibly fixate the external side of the ear with double-sided adhesive tape
  - Place a swab onto the internal side of the ear
  - Apply a cotton wool dressing that leaves the healthy ear out
  - Add an elastic gauze dressing
  - Possibly fixate the edges of the dressing to the fur with adhesive tape
  - Leave a space of two fingers width between collar and ventral neck

Complications

- Dressing might slip
- Otitis externa

Bilateral Ear Dressing

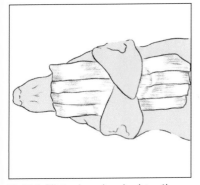

Fig 23.7 Bilateral ear dressing (step 1)

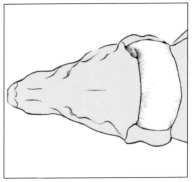

Fig 23.8 Bilateral ear dressing (step 2)

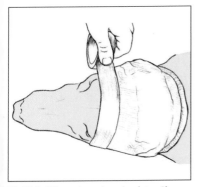

Fig 23.9 Bilateral ear dressing (step 3)

Method

- **Technique**
  - Place a wide adhesive strip onto the top of the head
  - Fold both ears onto adhesive strip
  - Fold the adhesive strip over
  - Apply stulpa head dressing (alternatively a pair of tights can be used)

Complications

- Dressing might slip
- Otitis externa

Corrective Dressing

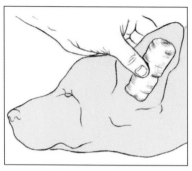

Fig 23.10 Unilateral corrective dressing (step 1)

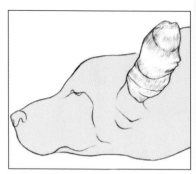

Fig 23.11 Unilateral corrective dressing (step 2)

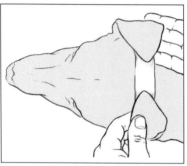

Fig 23.12 Bilateral corrective dressing (step 1)

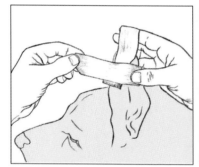

Fig 23.13 Bilateral corrective dressing (step 2)

Method

- **Technique**

  Unilateral
  - Place a gauze roll to the inside of the pinna
  - Apply an adhesive ear dressing

  Bilateral
  - Place two layers of adhesive dressing against each other to the inside and outside of each ear
  - Apply an adhesive ear dressing for each ear

Complications

- Dressing might slip

Head/Neck Dressing

Indication

- Wound dressing

Head/Neck Dressing

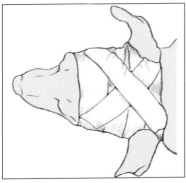

Fig 23.14 Head dressing

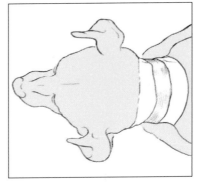

Fig 23.15 Neck dressing

Method

- **Technique**

    Head Dressing
    - Treat the wound
    - Apply a cotton wool dressing (in crossover pattern while leaving the ears outside of the dressing)
    - Apply an elastic gauze dressing
    - Possibly fixate the edges of the dressing to the fur with adhesive tape
    - Leave a space of two fingers width between the collar and the ventral neck

    Neck Dressing
    - Treat the wound
    - Apply a cotton wool dressing (in crossover pattern)
    - Apply an elastic gauze dressing
    - Fixate the edges of the dressing to the fur with adhesive tape
    - Leave a space of two fingers width between collar and ventral neck

Complications

- Dressing might slip off
- Breathing/swallowing difficulties

Thoracic Dressing

Indication

- Wound dressing
- Protective dressing (thoracic drainage)

Thoracic Dressing

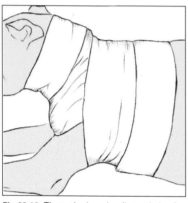

Fig 23.16 Thoracic dressing (lateral view)

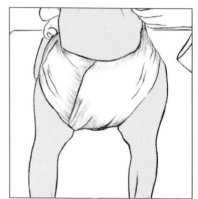

Fig 23.17 Thoracic dressing (cranial view)

Method

- **Technique**
  - Treat the wound
  - Apply a cotton wool dressing (crossover pattern)
  - Apply an elastic gauze dressing (crossover pattern)
  - Fixate the edges of the dressing to the fur with adhesive tape
  - Leave a space of two fingers width between the collar and the ventral neck

Complications

- Dressing might slip off
- Breathing difficulties

Abdominal Dressing

Indication

- Wound Dressing
- Protective Dressing (drains)

Abdominal Dressing

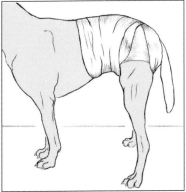

Fig 23.18 Abdominal dressing (lateral view)

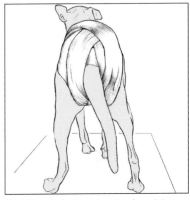

Fig 23.19 Abdominal dressing (caudal view)

Method

- **Technique**
  - Treat the wound
  - Apply a cotton wool dressing (crossover pattern) while leaving the body orifices out
  - Apply an elastic gauze dressing (crossover pattern) while leaving the body orifices out
  - Fixate the edges of the dressing to the fur with adhesive tape
  - Leave a space of two fingers width between collar and ventral neck

Complications

- Dressing might slip off
- Soiling

Tail Dressing

Indication

- Wound dressing
- Protective dressing

Tail Dressing

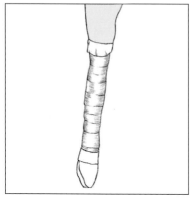

Fig 23.20 Padded tail dressing

Method

- **Technique**
  - Treat the wound
  - Cover the wound (gauze swab)
  - Apply an elastic gauze dressing (crossover pattern)
  - Fixate the edges of the dressing to the fur with adhesive tape

Complications

- Dressing might slip

Bandage for the Forelimb

Indication

- Wound dressing
- Protective dressing

Bandage for the Forelimb

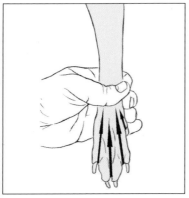

Fig 23.21 Padding of the toes with cotton wool

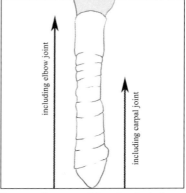

Fig 23.22 Cotton wool dressing (including elbow/carpal joint)

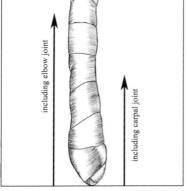

Fig 23.23 Elastic gauze dressing (including elbow/carpal joint)

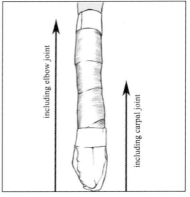

Fig 23.24 Adhesive tape dressing (including elbow/carpal joint)

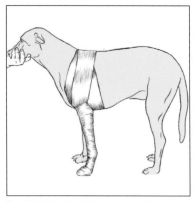

Fig 23.25 Forelimb/shoulder bandage

Method

- **Technique**
  - Treat the wound
  - Cover the wound (gauze swab)

Padding of the toes with cotton wool
  - Apply four cotton wool strips between the toes

Cotton wool dressing
  - Single/double pattern around the sole of the foot
  - Parallel pattern (overlay of the cotton wool strips by about 50 per cent) from the paw to proximal of the carpal joint/elbow joint

Elastic gauze dressing
  - Single/double pattern around the sole of the foot
  - Crossover pattern from the paw to proximal of the carpal/elbow joint

Adhesive tape dressing
  - Protection of the sole of the foot (four vertical strips and one transverse strip)
  - Fixate the edges of the gauze dressing to the fur

Complications

- Dressing might slip off
- Pressure necrosis
- Putrefaction
- Unaccepting/panic (especially cats)

Bandage for the Hind Limb

Indication

- Wound dressing
- Protective dressing (scratch protection)

Bandage for the Hind Limb

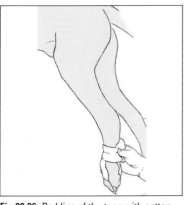

Fig 23.26 Padding of the toes with cotton wool

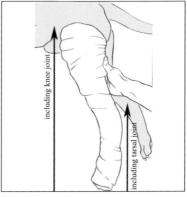

Fig 23.27 Cotton wool dressing (including knee/tarsal joint)

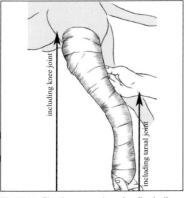

Fig 23.28 Elastic gauze dressing (including knee/tarsal joint)

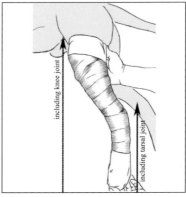

Fig 23.29 Adhesive tape dressing (including knee/tarsal joint)

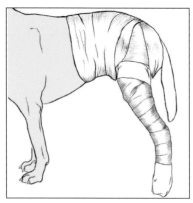

Fig 23.30 Bandage of the hind limb with abdominal dressing

Method

- **Technique**
  - Treat the wound
  - Cover the wound (gauze swab)

Padding of the toes with cotton wool

  - Apply four cotton wool strips between the toes

Cotton wool dressing

  - Single/double pattern around the sole of the foot
  - Parallel pattern (overlay of the cotton wool strips by about 50 per cent) from the paw to proximal of the tarsal/knee joint

Elastic gauze dressing

  - Single/double pattern around the sole of the foot
  - Crossover pattern from the paw to proximal of the tarsal/knee joint

Adhesive tape dressing

  - Protection of the sole of the foot (four vertical strips and one transverse strip)
  - Fixate the edges of the gauze dressing to the fur

Complications

- Dressing might slip off
- Pressure necrosis
- Putrefaction
- Unaccepting/panic (especially cats)

Elbow Dressing

Indication

- Wound dressing
- Protective dressing

Elbow Dressing

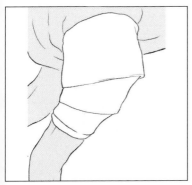

Fig 23.31 Wound dressing/cotton wool dressing

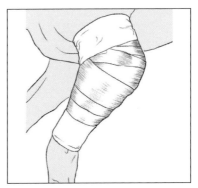

Fig 23.32 Elastic gauze dressing/adhesive tape dressing

Method

- **Technique**
  - Treat the wound
  - Cover the wound (gauze swab)
  - Cotton wool dressing
  - Crossover pattern (from distal to proximal of the elbow joint)
  - Elastic gauze dressing
  - Crossover pattern (from distal to proximal of the elbow joint)
  - Adhesive tape dressing
  - Fixate the edges of the elastic gauze dressing to the fur

Complications

- Dressing might slip off
- Pressure necrosis
- Swelling of the distal limb

Stifle Dressing

Indication

- Wound dressing
- Protective dressing

Stifle Dressing

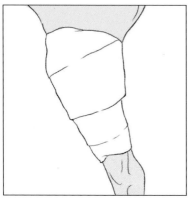

Fig 23.33 Wound dressing/cotton wool dressing

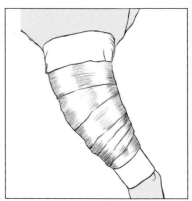

Fig 23.34 Elastic gauze dressing/adhesive tape dressing

Method

- **Technique**
  - Treat the wound
  - Cover the wound (gauze swab)

  Cotton wool dressing
  - Crossover pattern (from distal to proximal of the stifle joint)

  Elastic gauze dressing
  - Crossover pattern (from distal to proximal of the stifle joint)

  Adhesive tape dressing
  - Fixate the edges of the gauze dressing to the fur

Complications

- Dressing might slip off
- Pressure necrosis
- Swelling of the distal limb

Robert-Jones Dressing

Indication

- Support dressing in acute limb trauma (fractures)

Robert-Jones Dressing

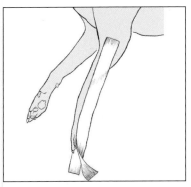

Fig 23.35 Stirrups of adhesive tape

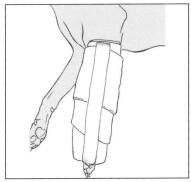

Fig 23.36 Cotton wool dressing

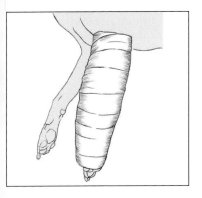

Fig 23.37 Elastic gauze dressing

Method

- **Technique**
  - Place the adhesive stirrups on the unshaved fur
  - Apply a generous sized cotton wool dressing leaving the paw out
  - Turn the stirrups over and adhere them to the cotton wool dressing
  - Add a tight gauze dressing

Elastic Bandage

Indication

- Support Dressing

Elastic Bandage

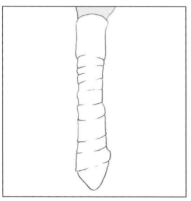

Fig 23.38 Padding of the toes with cotton wool/cotton wool dressing

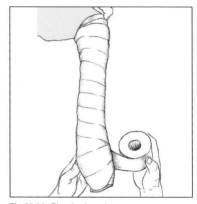

Fig 23.39 Elastic dressing

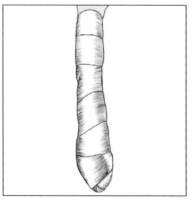

Fig 23.40 Elastic gauze dressing

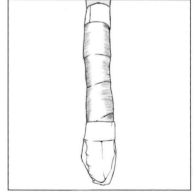

Fig 23.41 Adhesive tape dressing

Method

- **Technique**
  - Treat the wound
  - Cover the wound (gauze swab)

  Padding of the toes with cotton wool
  - Apply four cotton wool strips between the toes
  - Cotton wool dressing
  - Single/double pattern around the sole of the foot
  - Parallel pattern (overlay of the cotton wool strips by about 50 per cent) from the paw to proximal of the elbow/knee joint

  Elastic dressing
  - Tight parallel pattern of elastic dressing

  Elastic gauze dressing
  - Single/double pattern around the sole of the foot
  - Crossover pattern from the paw to proximal of the elbow/stifle joint

  Adhesive tape dressing
  - Protection of the sole of the foot (four longitudinal adhesive strips and one transverse one)
  - Fixate the edges of the gauze dressing on the fur

Complications

- Swelling
- Pressure necrosis
- Putrefaction
- Unacceptance/panic (especially cat)

Splint Bandage

Indication

- Support dressing for immobilisation of the limb

Synthetic Casting Tape

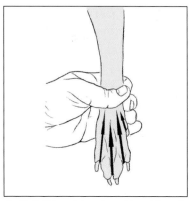

Fig 23.42 Wound dressing with padding of the toes

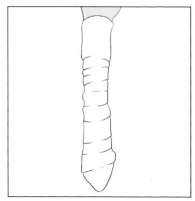

Fig 23.43 Cotton wool dressing

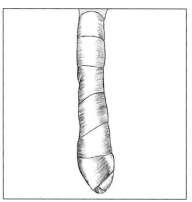

Fig 23.44 Elastic gauze dressing

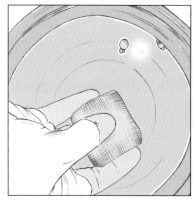

Fig 23.45 Knead the cast in lukewarm water

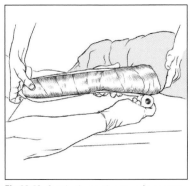

Fig 23.46 Synthetic casting tape (measure the length)

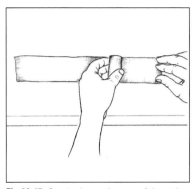

Fig 23.47 Synthetic casting tape (place the straps)

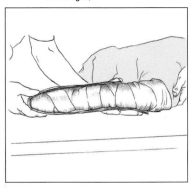

Fig 23.48 Synthetic casting tape (application)

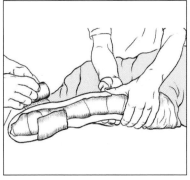

Fig 23.49 Elastic gauze dressing

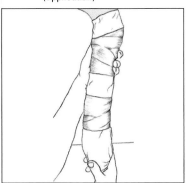

Fig 23.50 Adhesive tape dressing

Method

- **Technique**
  - Treat the wound
  - Cover the wound (gauze swab)

Padding of the toes with cotton wool
  - Place four cotton wool strips between the toes

Cotton wool dressing
  - Single/double pattern around the sole of the foot
  - Parallel pattern (overlay of the cotton wool strips by about 50 per cent) from the paw to proximal of the elbow/knee joint

Elastic gauze dressing
  - Single/double pattern around the sole of the foot
  - Crossover pattern from the paw to proximal of the elbow/stifle joint

Synthetic casting tape
  - Cellacast Xtra®, Lohmann & Rauscher
  - Knead for 1 min in lukewarm water wearing gloves
  - Measure the required length on the patient
  - Fold the tape in overlaying strips and lay onto a table or plastic work top
  - Brush the dressing surface with a greasy cream
  - Apply the dressing
  - Adapt it to the shape of the limb
  - Round the edges off and turn them outwards (pair of dressing scissors as required)

Elastic gauze dressing
  - Single/double pattern around the sole of the foot
  - Crossover pattern from the paw to proximal of the synthetic casting tape

Adhesive tape dressing
  - Protection of the sole of the foot (four longitudinal adhesive strips and one transverse one)
  - Fixate the edges of the gauze dressing on the fur

Complications

- Swelling
- Pressure necrosis
- Putrefaction
- Unacceptance/panic (esp. cat)

Schröder-Thomas Dressing

Indication

- (Obsolete) support dressing for tibia/radius and ulna fractures

Schröder-Thomas Dressing

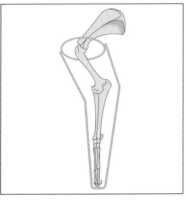

Fig 23.51 Schröder-Thomas splint
(forelimb)

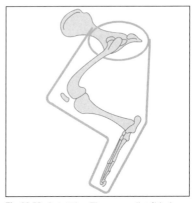

Fig 23.52 Schröder-Thomas splint (hind
limb)

Method

- **Technique**
  - Treat the wound
  - Cover the wound (gauze swab)
  - Apply a gauze dressing
  - Pre-bend the splint (oval aluminium tube 1.5 turns + U-shaped tube)
  - Pad the tube
  - Apply the splint

  Gauze tension dressing
  - Femur (paw: distal tension, metatarsalia: posterior tension, femur: anterior tension)
  - Humerus (paw: distal tension, humerus: posterior tension)

Complications

- Rotation
- Pressure necrosis

Ehmer-Sling Bandage

Indication

- Relief dressing following reposition of the hip joint

Ehmer-Sling Bandage

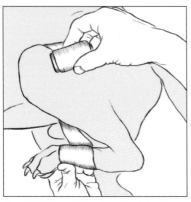

Fig 23.53 Ehmer-Sling direction (step 1)

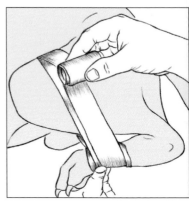

Fig 23.54 Ehmer-Sling direction (step 2)

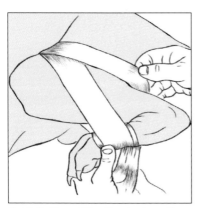

Fig 23.55 Ehmer-Sling direction (step 3)

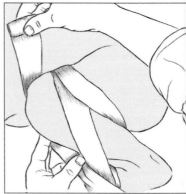

Fig 23.56 Ehmer-Sling direction (step 4)

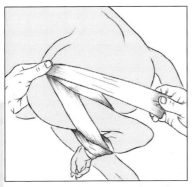

Fig 23.57 Ehmer-Sling direction (step 5)

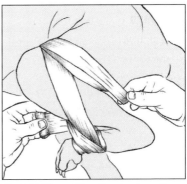

Fig 23.58 Ehmer-Sling direction (step 6)

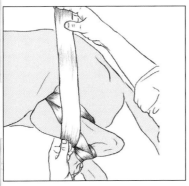

Fig 23.59 Ehmer-Sling direction (step 7)

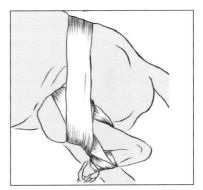

Fig 23.60 Ehmer-Sling direction (step 8)

Method

- **Technique**
  - Gauze dressing/adhesive tape dressing
  - Sling direction 1–8

Complications

- Dressing might slip off
- Unacceptance

Velpeau-Sling Bandage

Indication

- Relief dressing after reposition of the shoulder joint/scapular fractures

Velpeau-Sling Bandage

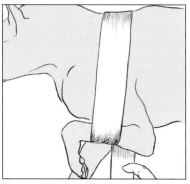

Fig 23.61 Velpeau-Sling (Step 1)

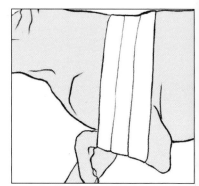

Fig 23.62 Velpeau-Sling (Step 2)

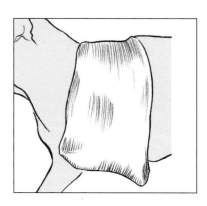

Fig 23.63 Velpeau-Sling (Step 3)

Method

- **Technique**
  - Gauze dressing/adhesive tape dressing

Complications

- Dressing might slip off
- Unacceptance

Robinson-Sling Bandage

Indication

- Relief Dressing of a hind limb

Robinson-Sling Bandage

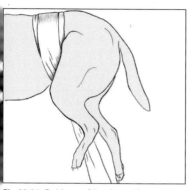

Fig 23.64 Robinson-Sling (step 1)

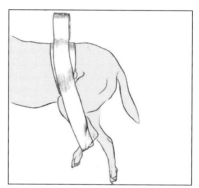

Fig 23.65 Robinson-Sling (step 2)

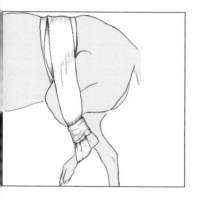

Fig 23.66 Robinson-Sling (step 3)

Method

- **Technique**
  - Gauze dressing/adhesive tape dressing

Complications

- Dressing might slip off

Hoppel-Sling Bandage

Indication

- Relief dressing after pelvic trauma (distal bandage)
- Relief dressing following reposition of the hip joint (proximal bandage)

Hoppel-Sling Bandage

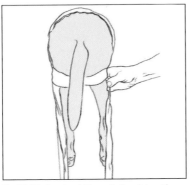

Fig 23.67 Proximal Hoppel sling (step 1)

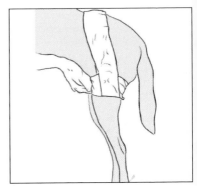

Fig 23.68 Proximal Hoppel sling (step 2)

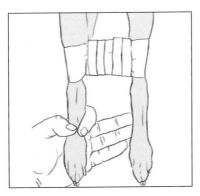

Fig 23.69 Distal Hoppel sling

Method

- **Technique**
  - Gauze dressing/adhesive tape dressing

Complications

- Dressing might slip off

Index